Praise for *Covid Vaccine Adverse*

'As a clinician working with those w ....jured by the Covid 19 vaccine, I am forever grateful for this book. At a time where many people have been ignored and silenced, and had their physical symptoms blamed on mental health conditions, this book is the go to guide for so many sufferers. Many medical doctors did not recognise vaccine injuries and worse, many sufferers were ridiculed and demonised for simply speaking their truth. Unfortunately, this led to the injured often having to take control of their health on their own. This is why Caroline Pover's guide is life-changing for many people.

Vaccine harm straddles both a physical and psychological injury. The physical injury itself is traumatic and we know that trauma can bring a wide range of emotional difficulties such as intrusive thoughts and imagery, hyper vigilance, feelings of anxiety and depression, and for some suicidal thinking. However, on top of this, many sufferers entire lives became instantly and significantly changed for the worse. Many cannot work, which brings financial hardship, relationships often break down due to a loss of identity, some have been terrified of not being believed or of being abused so have hidden away from society for fear of judgment. These feelings in conjunction with the trauma experienced as a direct result of the physical injury can easily contribute to feelings of hopelessness. In my job as a psychotherapist, hopelessness is one of my biggest enemies and one of the most significant warning signs. This book provides hope for so many people. Alongside the support group of UKCVFamily, this guide gives that glimmer of hope desperately needed by many, and proves to suffers who feel no one cares and they are on their own, that, actually, there are thousands and thousands of people struggling just like them and that there are many, many good people who do care.

Caroline is the expert by experience, and her knowledge is shared in this amazing book. Whether you are injured yourself, know someone who has been injured, or just want to understand more about helping those who are injured, this guide is the "must have" book on surviving Covid 19 vaccine adverse reactions.'

Dr Christian Buckland
Psychotherapist and psychological advisor to UKCVFamily

Covid Vaccine Adverse Reaction Survival Guide

Covid Vaccine Adverse Reaction Survival Guide

Take Control of Your Recovery and Maximise Healing Potential

Understand the Practical and Emotional Impact of your Symptoms
and Learn to Organise Every Step of your Health Management

CAROLINE POVER

Chelsea Green Publishing
London, UK
White River Junction, Vermont USA

Commissioning Editor: Brianne Goodspeed
Project Manager: Laura Jones
Design and page layout: Caroline Pover
Editor and Proofreader: Cindy Fujimoto
Proofreader: Jacqui Lewis
Cover design: Caroline Pover with Dexter Fry
Author photo: ©571Photography (Ian Lloyd-Graham)

First edition published by Caroline Pover in 2021.
This edition published by Chelsea Green Publishing in 2023.

Printed in the United States of America.
First printing September 2023.
10 9 8 7 6 5 4 3 2 1   23 24 25 26 27

ISBN 978-1-915294-26-5 (paperback)
ISBN 978-1-915294-27-2 (ebook)

Chelsea Green Publishing
London, UK
White River Junction, Vermont USA

www.chelseagreen.co.uk

For Sandie

CONTENTS

MY STORY

On March 3rd, 2021 at 12:20pm I was given one dose of AstraZeneca's Covid vaccine. I didn't even feel the needle go in.

Nine hours later, I started shaking. Full body shakes. And I was freezing cold. My teeth were chattering loudly. I looked down at my hands to find them violently shaking — I had never experienced anything like this before. I got into bed fully clothed and put the electric blanket on high. By 2am I was still shaking and my cognitive functions were no longer working properly. My boyfriend called an ambulance, and the paramedics ascertained that my vitals were at dangerous levels so they took me into A&E, stabilising me on the way. I had numerous scans and blood tests, none of which gave any clues as to what was happening to me. I was discharged the next day with a diagnosis of "Severe reaction to Covid vaccine."

I had no idea that vaccines could cause this kind of reaction. I had never heard of a severe reaction to any kind of vaccine. I actually questioned the diagnosis.

In the days that followed I slept for hours, having vivid, disturbing dreams the likes of which I have never experienced either before or since. I was constantly exhausted, able to do little more than shower. My chest was tight and breathing was difficult, and I developed a huge, stinging rash from my vulva all the way up my back, then unexpectedly started menstruating. After that, the migraines started — daily migraines accompanied by numbness on one side of my face, my tongue, my arm, or my leg, and a complete loss of awareness of where I was or who I was with. Sometimes I hallucinated. I felt like I'd had a stroke.

Exactly a week after the vaccine I experienced excruciating head pain that had me in tears, convinced that if I stuck a knife in the side of my head that would somehow relieve the pain. Painkillers made no difference whatsoever. Another ride in an ambulance resulted in the same diagnosis: "Severe reaction to Covid vaccine." I found out almost two years later that I was actually diagnosed with a stroke. Nobody told me at the time.

I was supposed to be launching my fifth book — a memoir — and had twenty speaking engagements lined up. I was writing another book, running a successful pickling business, learning Japanese, doing yoga every day, and regularly running or hiking. I was leading a busy, fulfilling life and suddenly I could no longer function. I cancelled everything.

In the following weeks I developed a range of weird physical and psychological symptoms. Every single day was different. I was in constant pain. Everything exhausted me — I couldn't even talk to anyone for long. I had to rest in bed after sleeping, showering, walking down the stairs, moving from one room to another. I had no idea what was going on. I knew nobody else that this had happened to. And nobody was helping me.

I created my own recovery plan, focusing on a "brain-food" diet and sleep — lots and lots of sleep. I got support from a counsellor, a Functional Medicine practitioner, and an acupuncturist, all of whom became my life-savers. My GP got on board with my recovery efforts — there was nothing she could do but she was at least kind and sympathetic. She insisted that I apply for a medical exemption, and always made extra time available to speak to me. In that regard I know that I was one of the lucky ones.

I eventually connected with other people from all over the world who were also dealing with adverse reactions to *all* of the Covid vaccines, not just AstraZeneca. I even connected with people who had experienced adverse reactions after participating in the trials. Nobody was getting any treatment, and very few people were getting any better. I planned on dedicating three months to my recovery — I was a big believer in the power of food as medicine, and I had faith in the body's natural ability to heal. I assumed that I would be back to normal after three months.

More than two years later, at the time of writing this revised section to the Chelsea Green edition, I am still not "back to normal." I have a new normal now.

I initially spent five months on full-time, intense recovery efforts before I began to see some glimpses of my old life. The game changer for me was the accidental discovery of therapeutic phlebotomy and the temporary relief that it brings —

perhaps there was something in that old bloodletting after all. It allowed me to experience little moments of joy occasionally, and gave me just a bit of energy so that I could go for a walk sometimes. I watched the world open up again and tried to participate in it, but instead found myself in an intensely divided and very *ugly* world seemingly defined by whether you were vaccinated or not, and I wasn't sure where I belonged in that. Or whether I even wanted to.

During the following seventeen months I continued with regular therapeutic phlebotomy, each time trying to make the most of the temporary life the treatment gave me — getting countless of tests done, exploring all sorts of different treatments, and spending thousands of pounds to try to get better. My savings disappeared so I launched a healthcare fund, and was touched by the kindness of people from all over the world who were following my journey and wanted me to recover.

I was also disheartened by people all over the world who were making a fortune out of a desperately sick and vulnerable community that had nowhere to turn. Or turning themselves into "Covid celebrities" all over social media with their unfounded claims to be curing us. When I get contacted about the latest "cure," I still today ask myself, who is the loudest about that cure — is it actually a patient or just another practitioner?

People forget — those of us with adverse reactions are the ones learning the most about them.

I tried to share everything I was learning. Not just about the different treatments or ways of looking at health that I had no idea existed, but also about how to manage a complex condition like this. I posted regularly on my social media, and still do, especially on my Facebook page, which you're more than welcome to explore. I started giving speeches and interviews about life through the lens of the vaccine-injured.

I became known for my commitment to healing myself, for communicating with a compassionate voice, and for trying to find humour in the middle of all of this. Then I suddenly and unexpectedly ended up in hospital with appendicitis. I very reluctantly had surgery, which turned into sepsis. It set me back months. I felt like I had during the early weeks post-vaccine. I was utterly devastated. I had worked so hard. I didn't have any fight left in me.

A one-way ticket to Switzerland felt like my only hope, and I started making plans. I told all the people closest to me and they didn't blame me one bit — they knew this wasn't the life that the Caroline they knew ever wanted to live. At least it was something I could look forward to.

I didn't end up going to Switzerland. I spent a few months allowing my body to settle after the distressing hospital experience, got back to where I was just before it, and unexpectedly discovered another game changer — copper — and overnight got more of my life back. A couple of months later there was another game changer — the 2pm sleep — and again, overnight, I got even more of my life back. Two such simple things made such a huge difference.

In the past six months I have gone from functioning at about a third of a reasonable life, to functioning at about double that. It requires constant management — if I miss a phlebotomy session, run out of copper, or don't sleep enough then I relapse very quickly. On most days I am now able to go on a short walk and have a 30-minute conversation with someone but if I need or want to do more than that then I need to plan days to recover. Managing my limitations and being patient with myself are my new normal.

I have no idea whether I will "fully" recover from this experience — I'm not entirely sure what my definition of "recovery" is right now. My life will never be what it was, and I am learning that, in some ways, it might even be better. The friendships I have made through this experience feel like deep connections with special souls that were all sent to help each other along the way during a unique time in our history.

I have personally found healing through spiritual, nutritional, and traditional means rather than pharmaceutical, but we are all different and what works for me might not feel right for you. This book is not about how I am surviving this — it's about helping you to survive it.

Caroline Pover
June, 2023

WHY I WROTE THIS BOOK

In the early weeks, I genuinely thought I was the only person in the world experiencing this kind of reaction to the vaccine. I couldn't find any information that would explain what was happening, or why, or how to deal with it. I was not getting any support from the medical professionals I turned to for help. I felt terribly alone, and wondered whether I was going insane.

Eventually, I plucked up the courage to post something on my Facebook page about what was happening to me, and was amazed to receive private messages from friends who were experiencing the same thing, but not saying anything. Then strangers started reaching out to me, and I discovered support groups that were sprouting up on social media, filled with thousands of people, from all over the world. I wasn't alone after all. And I wasn't going insane.

I couldn't bear the thought of anybody feeling as isolated as I did during those early weeks, so I started regularly posting about what was happening to me, including the efforts I was taking in my own recovery. I joined some of the support groups and tried to give more than I took. People from around the world started following my personal page, and I was invited to become an admin on one of the support groups. A few months later, that support group was shut down, and it became apparent that not only were many medical professionals unable or unwilling to help us, but the ways we were creating to help *ourselves* were being threatened.

I spent fifteen years running my own independent publishing company in Japan, and I have independently published my own books as well as other people's. It was a natural step for me to put together all the different things I have learned in a format that I am so comfortable with — one that cannot be censored or silenced.

Helping others has been a theme throughout my whole life. I hope that the tools I have developed for my own recovery during the past year will help you.

DISCLAIMERS & DISCLOSURES

I have no medical training or qualifications whatsoever. I have never been on any kind of healthcare course. I am not affiliated with any individual or organisation related to healthcare. I have no financial interest in any medical products.

For the purposes of transparency, I studied Mathematics and Education at Exeter University in the UK, and graduated with a First Class Honours degree and a Dean's Commendation. I am a qualified primary school teacher, but have not taught for over 25 years. I am an entirely self-taught writer, publisher, and food producer. I ran my own publishing company for fifteen years. I currently run a food business. I have a Food Hygiene certificate related to my food business — not at all related to healthcare. The numerous awards I have received for writing, speaking, entrepreneurship, and philanthropy are also not at all related to healthcare.

This book contains things I have learned as part of my own personal recovery journey. I have tried not to give specific advice because we are all unique and what is working for me may not work for you. I do not suggest ways we can "get fixed" because there aren't any right now. But we do have ways to manage our situation: ways of keeping track of appointments, tests, and the thoughts we all have; and ways of trying not to become overwhelmed by the whole process. Disclaimers like this usually advise readers to consult with their doctors before following advice, but how can we consult with them if they refuse to acknowledge what's happening to us? Hopefully you get my point — use this book at your own risk.

HOW TO USE THIS BOOK

I strongly advise that you work through this book slowly. Resist the urge to read all the way through right away — there's a lot of information here and it might be easy to feel overwhelmed by it. Take it one chapter at a time, and don't rush through any of them. Give yourself time to let the concepts sink in — much of this book is about spending time examining our current attitudes toward healthcare, recovery, and healing in general. It's possible that you might find yourself feeling resistant toward certain sections in this book because they cause you to want to make some uncomfortable or scary changes within yourself. Just sit with those feelings for a while until you feel ready to look at that particular section with perhaps a more open heart and mind. Healing is a difficult process that requires internal reflection and the ability to be patient with ourselves.

I recommend that you work through the book in the order in which it is presented. For example, work through the Sleep chapter first, then the Food chapter, and so on. I deliberately wrote this book in the order of what I feel are the priorities that anyone would have when recovering from any kind of physical or emotional trauma, and that first priority is always sleep. You can go to the best specialists in the world, but their advice won't be half as effective if you're not getting good quality sleep every night, and plenty of it. I suggest that you really get to grips with a single chapter, implement what feels relevant to you in your daily life, and make those changes habitual before moving on to the next chapter — you don't need to do everything at once. Again: patience is key.

Having said all that, if you just want to use the book as something you can dip in and out of, depending on what's bothering you the most, then by all means go ahead. Just know that it is designed to be worked through bit by bit, slowly.

The Wheel of Healing is something that you can use directly in the book, but it's also something you can easily sketch and stick on your fridge or wherever is the most helpful for you. It is a wheel because while there may be a very clear beginning to our healing process, the "end" isn't quite so clear. The Wheel of Healing is intended to acknowledge the non-linear nature of healing, as well as promote the idea of us moving *forward*, but at our own pace. Even if we find ourselves dealing with something more than once, we are still moving forward.

Each of the six sections of the wheel is intended to give you space to note one or two elements of your recovery that pertain to each chapter: Sleep, Food, Symptoms, Stress, Consultants, and Connections. Your Wheel of Healing will change throughout your recovery — the things you choose to focus on during the first month might be very different from what you feel you need to focus on around month six. There is a blank Wheel of Healing at the back of the book.

There are also some blank weekly, monthly, and annual diaries at the back of the book that might help you organise your recovery as well as give you a way of reflecting on how far you've come. You don't have to use these, but they are helpful tools if you feel you want to try them. And you never know how useful they may be further down the line when meeting new consultants, or even for any legal steps you might decide to look into.

This book is designed for you to write in it, wherever is helpful for you. Fill in the charts, highlight bits that appeal to you — do whatever you need to do to make this your own. Although my publisher and I have also produced a digital edition to make the book as widely available as possible, I am reluctant to encourage you to spend more time in front of screens — we end up doing enough of that as we research medical information and online support groups. In general, do as much as you can offline, away from a screen, and use a pen or pencil with this book, the old-fashioned way.

Finally, how *not* to use this book ...

This is not a book that will give you any quick fixes or easy answers. There is no quick fix to recovery, and no one seems to have any real answers when it comes to recovering from an adverse reaction to the Covid vaccine. This book is a *tool* to help you take charge of your recovery. It is not a book about cures or magical answers to make all your symptoms disappear. It is a *survival guide* — a way to get through it.

Before you start this chapter ...

Take a moment to think about how you feel about your sleep at the moment. What was your sleep pattern before the vaccine? How about in the days that followed? How are you sleeping now? How do you feel when you wake up? Do you feel that you are getting enough sleep? Use the space above to make note of any of your thoughts or feelings about sleep, especially in relation to life since the vaccine.

CHAPTER 1: SLEEP

SUMMARY

Your brain is repairing while it sleeps.
Sleep needs to become a priority.
Spend time preparing for sleep.
Sleep as long as you need to (no alarm).
Find opportunities to sleep during the day.
Congratulate yourself for getting lots of sleep.

We all know that sleep is probably the most important thing for us when we're recovering from any illness. In "normal" times, sleep gives our bodies and brains the opportunity to recharge after the day's activities. We know when we've had enough sleep because we wake up feeling refreshed and energised — ready for another day. Our brains and bodies are recharged. But for many of us dealing with an adverse reaction, our sleep is greatly disrupted, so that recharging just isn't happening at a time when we really, really need it.

Whether it's struggling to get to sleep or waking up throughout the night, we don't seem to be able to get the quality or quantity of sleep that we need in order to create a good foundation for our recovery. And when we do sleep, we don't wake up feeling refreshed. Our body's rhythm has been completely thrown out of sync, so we're not giving our brains and bodies the most basic thing they need to repair.

Getting ourselves back into sync is something that requires significant effort, but it's essential for us to get on top of our sleep, first and foremost, so that we can deal with more specific physical, cognitive, or emotional problems brought about by the adverse reaction. We need to start seeing sleep as our best friend and find ways that we can have as much of it as possible in our lives.

Adjusting Our Routine

In order to get more sleep — both quality and quantity — we will probably need to make some significant changes to our routines, which might be influenced by our finances, living situations, families, jobs, and any other responsibilities we may have. If we're honest, we might not even have been getting enough sleep before the vaccine anyway, so some big changes may need to be made, maybe even to accommodate sleeping during the day if you feel you are able and need to.

Most of us tend to be *really* good at creating excuses for not having enough sleep, or for telling ourselves that there are all sorts of obstacles that get in the way of us going to bed earlier or sleeping for longer. We can't use those excuses or obstacles now — sleep has become too important to us. We need to look for solutions, so let's get those excuses out of the way.

Sleep Obstacles	
What obstacle is stopping me from getting more sleep?	How can I remove that obstacle?

The Active Sleep Process

We may not have ever needed to think about what is actually involved in the process of "getting to sleep" before. We tend to think of it as something that just naturally happens (or doesn't), and is rather out of our control. If we're struggling with sleep and are looking at ways to adjust our routine to accommodate more of it, then it might help to increase our awareness of the entire process. I found it really helpful to think about these three different elements to my sleep patterns and new sleep needs:

- How I actively prepare for sleep.
- How I gently ease out of sleep.
- How I take opportunities to sleep during the day.

Sleep Preparation

Preparing for sleep does not always come naturally to many of us, and it's an essential habit to cultivate as we recover. I recommend spending a couple of hours actually preparing for sleep — it doesn't have to all be done in bed, but definitely spend the last hour there. During this time, focus on trying to calm your brain and send it messages that you're going to switch off soon. There are lots of techniques you can try before you find a routine that works for you. Here are some things that have worked for me ...

- **No "active" movies:** I might watch some *Friends* reruns on the TV in the living room, but I don't watch anything that requires me to concentrate or anything that is especially stimulating either visually or psychologically in the evening.
- **A sleep alarm:** Literally an alarm on my phone to tell me when to start getting ready for sleep. I set this for 30 minutes before I want to be in bed (not 30 minutes before I want to be asleep).
- **No screens before bed:** After that alarm goes off so do any screens that might be on (computer, TV, phone). And I don't keep my phone in the bedroom.
- **Bedtime drinks:** I have either some warm coconut milk with cacao, cinnamon, or turmeric; or fresh lemon, honey, and grated ginger steeped in hot water; or chamomile or peppermint tea.
- **A bath:** I've been using Epsom salts — the magnesium in the salt is supposed to be beneficial for detoxing and for pain and headaches in general. Having lived in Japan for fifteen years, I'm a

fan of the hot springs there, and you can now get "onsen powder" online, which is also believed to have healing properties.

- **Sleep hypnosis:** I found Paul McKenna's sleep hypnosis materials (search online) to be a life-saver during the first couple of months after the vaccine. (I needed my phone in the bedroom to be able to listen to him but, once I'd overcome my need for the hypnosis, I didn't bring it into the bedroom anymore.)

- **Diaphragm breathing:** A simple explanation — breathe in to a slow count to ten, but take very slow, deep breaths. When you think you've breathed in as much as you can, then breathe in some more; breathe right into your stomach until you feel your stomach push right out. Then breathe it all out again really, really slowly — keep pushing out even when you think there's nothing left. Do that over and over again.

- **Face massage:** Granted it's more relaxing if you can get someone else to give you a face massage, but it's *really* easy to do it yourself. Try gentle, sweeping movements all over your face with your fingertips, using just a little pressure, starting in the centre and moving outward or downward. Do this on your forehead, over your eyebrows, at the top and also the bottom of your eye sockets, along your sinuses, along your cheekbones, down your jawline, and down your chin.

- **Sex:** More specifically, an orgasm. It might be the last thing you feel like doing right now because you're so anxious, or maybe you're worried about heart palpitations, but I find the build-up to an orgasm to be a great way to take my mind away from worrying. It gets the happy part of the brain going, releases a flood of feel- good chemicals afterward, and promotes sleep. You obviously don't need a partner for it, but if you do have a partner, then you'll reconnect in a pure, deep, instinctual way that both of you might need right now. It's a good reminder that, despite everything you're dealing with, there is still joy to be found in life.

Those are the things that have worked, and still work, for me. Sleeping alone also helps, so, if your partner doesn't mind, ask to sleep alone once in a while ... although perhaps not after they've just, ahem, helped you prepare for sleep, which might be a bit insulting! I've gone through different phases where some things have worked better than others, and it probably took me about four months to get to the point where I was sleeping enough for both my body and my brain. I also had acupuncture specifically to help with sleeping. However, after about five months of having normal sleep again, I caught a mild cold that reactivated some of my vaccine symptoms, and I was back to square one with sleep again. It took about two months to reset to a healthy pattern. So you might need to be patient, and perhaps make the effort more than once. It will be worth it.

Have a think about all the different ways you can actively prepare your body for sleep, and keep track of which ones work best for you. Don't expect to see immediate results.

Actively preparing for sleep	
Things to try	How they're working for me

Gently Easing Out of Sleep

I found very early on that, even if I thought I had the energy to get up quickly, my body really did not like that *at all*, so I had to learn how to ease myself gently into the day.

I don't set an alarm. Ever. Still now, a year on, I allow my body to sleep as much as it needs to (it's now about ten hours a night) and, if I think I might be woken by anything other than my body's natural readiness to wake, then I plan for that, such as by wearing earplugs or an eye mask. And nobody in my house *ever* disturbs me when I'm sleeping.

There are a whole range of reasons that might make it incredibly difficult to ease into your day gently, and we need to find our way around them somehow, especially during the early weeks and months when we might be needing up to double the amount of sleep that we used to get. We will need the cooperation and support of anyone else that lives with us, possibly our employers, and maybe our friends and family too, just to be able to prioritise sleep.

If you have a partner who doesn't usually take responsibility for the morning routine, now is the time for them to step up. If you have teenagers, they can organise themselves without your input. Come to think of it, most preteens can manage themselves if we've taught them how to. Plan it the day before, during one of your "pockets" of energy. And be kind to yourself — so your kids might not eat the healthiest food, they might wear odd socks and forget their homework for a while — it's really not the end of the world. They'll be learning other things, such as how to support someone who is sick, which I'd always argue is more valuable than some maths homework anyway. But, because not all schools will see it that way, let them know what's going on. You don't have to tell them that it's due to a vaccine if you don't want to have that conversation with them. Just tell them that you've come down with a sudden, unexplained, debilitating condition that your family is trying to adjust to.

If you have young kids and you're on your own, get help. Is there someone who can come and stay with you for a while? Ask friends, family, and neighbours if they can help you out. Do whatever it takes to get help managing your kids (or dog) in the morning so you can focus on sleeping for as long as you need to, and then ease yourself gently into the world each day.

Have a think about the things you can do to give yourself the time as well as the peace and quiet your body needs in order to maximise the benefits of nighttime sleep. Who do you need to communicate with in order to get support for a new morning routine? How can you ensure that you gently ease out of sleep?

Gently easing out of sleep	
Things I can change about my waking routine	How they're working for me

Opportunities for Daytime Sleeping

I was never one for so much as the teeniest snooze during the day, so I understand how hard it can be to even consider sleeping during the day as part of your routine. But I had to do it for *months* after the vaccine, and I do recommend it. I found that it allowed my brain to recover from any activity I'd just completed, and I think that it allowed more of my proper nighttime sleep to be devoted to repairing my brain.

For many of us dealing with an adverse reaction, the fatigue is *debilitating*. It feels like our bodies don't have enough energy to cope with recovering from the vaccine, let alone enough to cope with normal daily activities that we used to do without a thought. So we need to recharge after every activity. Sometimes that means sleeping, sometimes it means resting. Either way, it means taking time out *during the day* to allow our bodies and our brains to repair and recharge.

In the early months, I got into the habit of checking in with myself after every single task, just to see if I might benefit from a little snooze. My nature is to move quickly from one task to another, so it required a lot of effort and awareness for me to pause in between activities. I had to change the way I looked at my tasks so that I automatically took a break in between every one of them.

I also changed the way I looked at the head pains and pressure that I continued to have *months* after the vaccine. I started to see the pain and pressure as little signs that I really needed to stop, so I tried not to be annoyed by them and instead acknowledged that they were there to help me recover. Eventually, when I got a little sign that my brain wasn't happy, I resisted the urge to plough on through with whatever I was doing and instead just found a quiet place to lie down, close my eyes, and try to shut my brain off for a while. Then my goal became to have enough sleep during the day to prevent getting to the stage where a head pain or pressure told me to stop. We need to recharge *before* our battery gets low.

If you struggle to actually sleep during the day, or to switch your brain off from the worrying that we're all doing while dealing with these adverse reactions, then find a technique that works for you. Maybe you know how to meditate, or you have other ways to turn off your mind. In the months after the vaccine I actually started writing an erotic fiction novel for women. In all seriousness, it was a way to stimulate the joyful part of my brain at a time when I was desperately unhappy,

8

scared, and worried. I found that the location of the novel came alive in my mind, so I went to that imaginary place and focused on every detail of it. It helped me switch off all the worry and go into a little dreamlike snooze where my brain could fully recharge. After about an hour of that, I was ready to go (in more ways than one). It was actually really good fun!

Daytime sleeping	
Signs that I need to recharge during the day	
Extra opportunities to snooze during the day	
Things I can do to help myself sleep during the day	

When You're Too Tired to Work

If you're not taking time off work already, then you're going to need to in order to focus on your recovery, especially if you're just too tired to work. I have been self-employed for over 25 years, I have managed to create a career out of things that I absolutely *love* doing, I work really hard, and I always have done. I really *do* understand how difficult it is to admit that, for whatever reason, you're no longer able to work. I know the thought is scary, but if you try to push on through with normal life, and normal work, then you're going to delay your recovery.

At the very least, if at all possible, you need to be working from home and definitely on reduced hours. Ideally you won't be working at all for several months. If you're in a work situation where taking time off for being sick is an option, then take it and don't feel at all guilty. This is *not* your fault. If you're in a situation where you don't get paid sick leave, or you're self-employed, please do whatever you can to either take a break from work or reduce your workload. You'll need to dig into your savings, apply for a mortgage holiday, claim government benefits, or ask friends and family to keep you afloat for a while. Please don't let worrying about your job be something that hampers your health.

And once you do start to see your health improving, don't go rushing back to work. Take it slowly, and remember that you're not just trying to recover just to be able to get back to work. You're also trying to recover to be able to socialise, exercise, enjoy your home, spend time with loved ones, and do all the things that you cared about before this happened. Don't let work be the only thing that takes up all the energy you manage to reclaim after the effort you put into your recovery.

What I'm going to do when I don't have to sleep so much!

Making Sleep an Achievement!

You may be the kind of person who prides themselves on needing a relatively small amount of sleep yet manages to have a very productive day. Or the kind of person whose self-esteem is very much dependent on constantly achieving *something* or working your way through a to-do list (these are not criticisms ... that latter one is me!). If this resonates with you, then spending significant periods of time sleeping is going to be psychologically very, very challenging.

I *knew* that sleep was absolutely vital to my recovery, and I made that my priority in my recovery, yet, somehow, in the early days I would wake up, check what time it was, and instantly call myself a loser for sleeping so long. Whoa! What was I thinking in starting the day by telling myself off?! This is absolutely no way for us to talk to ourselves, especially if we're feeling vulnerable in any way. What would be the point in having all this great quality sleep if the first thing I do when I wake up is to make myself feel bad?

So I learned to embrace the hours of sleep I got. I congratulated myself on all the sleep I'd had, like it was a huge achievement. And this worked really well for me — it completely changed my feelings about needing to sleep so much.

I really want you to try to embrace sleep too. I'd love for you to wake up and literally tell yourself, "Well done for all that sleep! Wow! You worked so hard repairing your brain for eleven hours! You're amazing!" Say it out loud. Acknowledge all the sleep you got. Then carry the serenity of that sleep with you. Don't rush into your day. Enter your day slowly.

The most amount of sleep I've achieved in a 24-hour period is ...

My Sleep Diary

Use this diary to keep track of how your sleep progresses over time. You don't need to write much, and you don't need to do it every day. It takes time to develop new habits. Maybe just take a moment each week to jot down a sentence or two about what's going on with your sleep. It will be a great way to look back later and see how far you've come! There are other diary tools at the back of the book.

Sleep Diary	
Date	What's going on with my sleep?

Sleep Diary	
Date	What's going on with my sleep?

My Sleep Chart

Use this to see how the hours of sleep you are getting over a 24-hour period correlate to your symptoms. You don't need to use this every day. Just put a little dot or a cross at the end of any day where you've been more aware of your sleep, and see if you notice any changes. It might help you work out how much sleep you need to achieve optimum management of your symptoms.

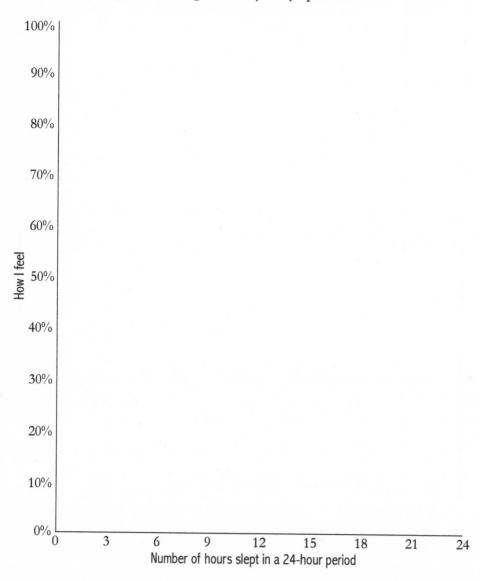

Wheel of Healing

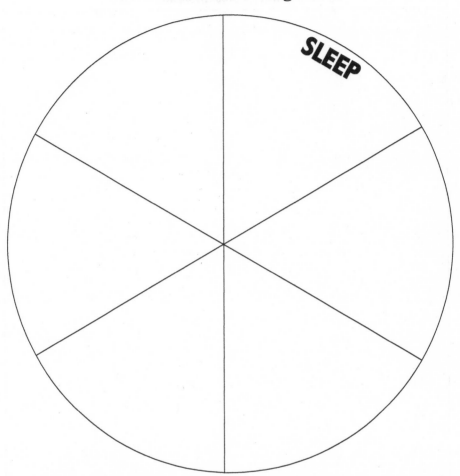

This "Wheel of Healing" will appear at the end of every chapter in the book, when it may be helpful to make a few notes regarding what you want to focus on at each stage in your recovery. As you go through the book, you will find that your attention to specific areas will change. For example, at some point you will be sleeping normally again (I promise!), so all you may need to note at that point is just to avoid late nights.

Make some notes in the Sleep section right now to remind yourself of what you're going to do to get your sleep not just back to a normal pattern, but to one that will maximise your body's ability to heal.

My Sleep Resources (books/websites/articles)

Other Notes/Thoughts on Sleep

Before you start this chapter ...

Take a moment to note what your normal diet is like. When do you eat? How often do you eat? What do you eat? Any restrictions? How often do you eat out? How often do you cook at home? How do you feel before, during, and after eating? How much liquid do you drink? And alcohol? Use the space above to make a note of any of your thoughts or feelings about food, both before and after the vaccine.

CHAPTER 2: FOOD

SUMMARY

Decide how important diet will be for your recovery.
Identify and cut out the things that will make you feel worse.
Add more foods that will boost your immune system.
Follow a targetted nutrition plan only IF it feels right for you.
Healing your gut will maximise the benefits of your food plan.
Setbacks can be learning opportunities.

There are three levels of intensity regarding how we can look at our diet when dealing with a vaccine injury.

- **Level One** is a pretty basic one, that I think all of us would agree with: try not to eat anything that makes us feel worse.
- **Level Two** involves generally improving our diet, and attempting to eat things that might help us feel a bit better in general.
- **Level Three** involves seeing food as medicine and following a targetted nutrition plan, perhaps with the support of a professional, with the specific purpose of maximising our body's ability to heal.

There are huge differences between each of these approaches, and they are not for everyone. Level Three involves an incredible amount of self-discipline and possibly access to financial resources, and, if you're not ready to embrace that entire way of living for at least several months, then it will just make you frustrated and miserable, which is going to result in the exact opposite of the intended effect. It can be easy to get caught up in worrying about whether you're eating the right or wrong food, and easy to be influenced by other people who seem to have completely mastered their diet in relation to their recovery.

It may seem like other people know exactly what they're doing when it comes to their diet but I can assure you that nobody does when it comes to an adverse reaction to the Covid vaccine. None of us *really* know what we're doing. We're all just making the best of our food decisions as we go along, with what limited knowledge we have, as we attempt to deal with an ever-changing health problem that is different for every single one of us.

You decide what level you feel comfortable with and capable of, and focus on that. Rest assured that your doing something, however small, will be better for your healing than doing nothing. You don't need to overcomplicate everything, especially in the early stages when it can be so easy to feel overwhelmed.

So let's keep it simple for now, and start with Level One — trying not to eat anything that makes us feel worse.

Level One: Food That Makes Us Feel Worse
Many of us suddenly find ourselves incredibly sensitive to food, whereas before the vaccine we may have been eating whatever we liked without any repercussions that we were aware of. Now, our immune systems are preoccupied and possibly compromised and confused by the vaccine — we appear to be displaying all the signs of a very high-level response to what our body perceives to be "invaders." Those presumed invaders seem to include some foods.

For many of us, some foods are suddenly triggering all sorts of intolerances or allergies that may not have been there before. We may find ourselves dealing with physical, cognitive, and psychological symptoms brought about by these new food intolerances, on top of other physical, cognitive, or psychological difficulties caused by further ways the vaccine may be impacting our body.

In order to minimise demands on our immune systems while they are still dealing with the vaccine, identifying what foods make us feel worse and avoiding or eliminating them from our diet is the first step in using food to help us recover. Foods that negatively impact our ability to heal generally include gluten, dairy, sugar, additives, and anything processed or preserved. Anything that isn't in a raw, pure form may create additional stress on the body through giving it extra elements to digest that your body isn't even going to use. Let's have a closer look at what might be making us feel worse.

Food that makes us feel worse			
Item	**What is it?**	**Where is it found?**	**Why might it make us feel worse?**
Gluten	Naturally occurring protein found in grains such as wheat and barley.	Breads, pastries, pies, pasta, pizza, imitation meats, beer, sauces.	Humans cannot digest it. Can trigger inflammation. Activates the immune system. Can lead to small intestine damage.
Dairy	Food produced from the milk of mammals.	Milk, cheese, cream, ice cream, butter, yoghurt.	Contains lactose, a type of sugar humans cannot digest.
Sugar	Sweet carbohydrates.	Occurs naturally in fruits and vegetables. Added to many foods.	Weakens the immune system.
Additives	Something added to a food to preserve or improve it.	Preservatives, colouring, artificial flavouring, flavour enhancers, stabilisers, thickeners.	Stresses the digestive system. Creates inflammation. Activates the immune system.
Processed Food	Any foods that have been altered during preparation.	Ready meals, frozen/tinned/dried/fermented foods, ground foods (like flour), cured meats, anything in a packet.	May lack nutrients. Creates inflammation. Affects healthy gut bacteria. Affects body's ability to detox. Weakens the immune system.

The idea of cutting all of the above out of your diet might seem very overwhelming, so just start slowly. Choose one item you feel comfortable cutting out, and focus on that for a month. You might be tempted to try for a few days then give up because you don't feel any different, but stick with it.

Whichever one you choose, you'll see an improvement in your health, and once you've done that, you might feel ready to eliminate something else, or even to take it to Level Two, and start looking at ways to incorporate certain foods into your diet as an attempt to continue feeling better.

Level Two: Generally Improving Our Diet

When we're looking at generally improving our diet, what we're really talking about for the purposes of dealing with an adverse reaction to the vaccine are ways to support our immune system.

What follows is intended to be a *very* simple overview of foods that will boost our immune system, plus some easy ways to add them to your existing diet without seeming too overwhelming to manage.

Food That Our Immune System Loves

Item	What it does	Easy ways to add it to our diet
Citrus fruits (oranges, lemons, limes, grapefruits)	Contains Vitamin C, which boosts the immune system. Also helps the body produce white blood cells, which fight off infection.	Juice and drink pure. Eat the fruit whole. Use instead of vinegar in cooking or dressings. Squeeze over green leafy veg (increases iron absorption too). Add hot/cold water to make a citrus drink.
Other fruits (especially papaya, kiwi, blueberries, pineapple, watermelon, apples, avocado, pomegranates)	Helps fight infections, protect cells, and aid digestion; helps with detoxing; maintains hydration; provides high levels of nutrients, and regulates blood pressure.	Apart from eating on their own (obviously) ... Make smoothies or non-dairy milkshakes. Juice. Add to porridge or non-dairy yoghurt. Warm up with non-dairy milk. Add to salads.
Vegetables (especially green leafy veg, red peppers, broccoli, spinach, garlic)	Helps fight infection, rich in vitamins, good for digestion.	Add to juice or smoothies. Incorporate in omelettes, salads. Steam as a side dish. Add to soups, curries, stir fries.
Whole grains (e.g., brown rice/bread/pasta)	Helps you retain nutrients; contains a fibre that boosts the immune system and helps reduces inflammation.	Switch refined rice/bread/pasta to whole grain.

Item	What it does	Easy ways to add it to our diet
Nuts and seeds	Helps blood flow. Contains Omega-3, zinc, and magnesium (boosts the immune system).	Sprinkle on salads. Eat nut/seed bread rather than normal bread. Spread nut/seed butter on a celery stick or carrot. Soak chia seeds in coconut milk/cream with berries.
Spices (especially ginger and turmeric)	Reduces inflammation, good for digestive health, prevents stress, helps repair damage.	Add to juices, smoothies, soups. Add to warm non-dairy milk. Make curries. Make salad dressing.
Live yoghurt	Contains beneficial bacteria for your gut, which helps fight infection and boosts the immune system.	Add to smoothies. Add to a fruit/nut/seed bowl. Add before serving curry or a Moroccan dish.
Probiotics (fermented foods)	Prevents overgrowth of unhelpful gut bacteria, reduces inflammation, protects cells.	Add sauerkraut/kimchi to salads. Add miso paste to soups. Drink kombucha/kefir. Add yoghurt to meals (see above).
Prebiotics	Promotes the growth of the good bacteria in your gut.	Add onions, leeks, garlic, apples, bananas, beans, peas, asparagus, artichokes.
Oily fish (especially salmon, mackerel, sardines)	Contains Vitamin A, reduces inflammation, enhances immune response.	Grill on toast. Flake on salads. Add to a soup. Serve with steamed vegetables.
Meat (especially chicken and turkey)	Contains Vitamin B6, which promotes white blood cell production.	Grilled/roasted and served with vegetables or in a curry/soup. Serve cold on a salad.
Bone broth	Repairs gut lining, helps with detoxing, reduces inflammation, reduces cell degeneration.	Cook vegetables/pasta/rice in it. Use as soup base. Drink as is.

Try to consume free-range, grass-fed, organic, homemade food, if you can, but honestly, I'm a bit of the mindset that any improvement is better than none, and it can't help us if we're worrying that our food doesn't meet those criteria.

The information on the preceding pages is intended to be a simple overview of things you can add to your existing diet that hopefully won't be too dramatic a change, and won't feel too overwhelming. The only exception to this might be the mention of bone broth, so if you're wondering what that is and how to go about getting it, let me reassure you that it is one of the *easiest* things to make, especially if you have a slow cooker. If you make bone broth a part of your daily diet, it's a very easy way to ramp up the immune-boosting potential of a lot of your meals.

Caroline's Really Easy Slow Cooker Bone Broth Recipe

Create a layer of vegetable scraps on the bottom of the slow cooker dish — anything will do: potato peelings, onion skins, carrot tops, beetroot leaves, etc. Sprinkle the vegetable scrap base with oregano, cayenne pepper, salt, and pepper. Place as many raw bones as you can on top of the vegetable base. Fill with water up to about an inch from the top. Splash cider vinegar in. Cook for 24 hours. Allow to cool slightly, then drain the liquid, and squish the final bits of liquid out of the vegetable scraps at the bottom. Cover and, when completely cooled, put it in the fridge. It will last about five days. After the first day the fat will have solidified on the top, and you can scrape it off and use it to make amazing roast potatoes. It's the gel-like liquid underneath that you want to keep (it will return to liquid when you reheat it).

You can use any bones, but I get the best results when I use lamb bones from the local sheep farmer, cooked from fresh.

The other simple way you can enhance the immune-boosting quality of your diet is by "eating the rainbow." This is based on the idea that eating colourful foods boosts the immune system, is good for the blood, and reduces inflammation. And it is so easy to implement. You aim for each meal to contain something red, orange, yellow, green, blue/purple, and white/brown/black. Need a red thing? Grill a tomato with those scrambled eggs. Orange? Grate some carrot over that salad. Yellow? Squeeze a lemon over wilted spinach or have a bit of pineapple. Green? Spread some avocado on that toast or have a few grapes. Blue/purple? Roast some beetroot with your turkey, or have a handful of blueberries. White/brown/black? Have a black coffee or a square of dark chocolate. There are lots of very simple ways to enhance your diet without having to go to the next level.

Level Three: Food as Medicine
This third approach is not for everyone, so if you've got this far, and just want to focus on cutting out anything that might be making you feel worse and adding a few things to boost your immune system, then that is absolutely FINE! You're doing great. Skim the rest of this chapter, get yourself a slow cooker, write your shopping list, experiment with some recipes, and focus on your healing. You can always come back to this if you feel you want to take it to the next level. You don't *have* to do everything in here or, indeed, *anything* anybody else suggests you do if it all feels a bit too much.

But, if you're of the mindset that food in itself can be a major part of your recovery programme, and you tend to be drawn more toward natural healing solutions rather than pharmaceutical, you might find yourself interested in what else you can do with your diet. Perhaps you've seen other people mention one diet or another that they're following and even having some success with, so you've started researching them yourself. The wonderful thing about the Internet is that all this information is just a click away, but the terrible thing about the Internet is that one click leads to another to another to another, and suddenly something that should be part of your healing now makes you feel even worse because it seems so complicated and absolutely impossible to incorporate into your life at a time when everything feels so overwhelming anyway.

So let's simplify all those food programmes that keep being mentioned in association with vaccine recovery.

On the following pages I have summarised a number of food regimes that are frequently referred to in the numerous adverse reaction communities online. I am sure you will recognise some of these, and perhaps have even tried some of them. As you look through these, perhaps one programme in particular will feel relevant to you. Perhaps a few of them will.

However, I recommend choosing just one to start with and then focusing on that one only, for a month. Often we try something new for just a few days, don't feel any different, and quickly lose motivation. We want results now! But it takes time for our bodies to heal and we need to be patient. Give whatever you try a full month to kick in. Remember — food is what fuels our body not just into action but into the creation of new cells, every single moment. That process takes time.

Anti-Inflammatory Diet	
Condition it deals with	Inflammation. Inflammation is when your body's immune system responds to infection caused by things like bacteria, viruses, or toxins. Signs of inflammation include heat, pain, redness, and swelling, which may be inside or on the surface of the body. These are signs that the body is producing cells or conducting activities aimed at reducing inflammation.
What the diet does	The Anti-Inflammatory Diet is aimed at reducing inflammation in the body. Foods consumed are intended to limit the effort required by the immune system, to fight off what it might perceive as threats. It is considered to reduce the levels of heat, pain, redness, and swelling throughout the body, and calm the immune system in general.
Why it might be relevant to us	Vaccines are designed to stimulate our body's response to infection. Some of us see visual evidence of redness, pain, or swelling as part of our adverse reactions, and some of us can feel those things happening inside our bodies. Some of us have blood test results that indicate inflammation is occurring. These are called inflammatory markers and might include erythrocyte sedimentation rate (ESR), C-reactive protein (CRP), and plasma viscosity (PV), but do not explain what has caused the inflammation. Some of us may have been dealing with inflammation throughout our body before the vaccine, but not known it, in which case the vaccine may have tipped our body's ability to deal with the inflammation beyond what it was able to deal with pre-vaccine.
Foods to avoid	Overly processed foods, fried foods, artificial trans fats (fats that have been processed e.g., margarine), vegetable and seed oils, refined carbohydrates (bread, pasta, cakes, etc.), processed meats (bacon, sausages), food additives, added sugars, excessive alcohol.
Helpful foods	FISH: tuna, salmon, mackerel, anchovies, halibut, trout, cod FRUIT: blueberries, blackberries, strawberries, cherries, oranges, apples, grapes, mangoes, peaches, bananas, pomegranates, dried fruits, lemons VEG: avocado, leafy greens (kale, spinach, lettuce, seaweed), broccoli, sprouts, cauliflower, tomatoes, peppers, garlic NUTS & SEEDS: walnuts, almonds, chia seed, flaxseed, sunflower seeds HERBS & SPICES: ginger, turmeric, cinnamon, cardamom, rosemary DRINKS: chamomile tea, coconut milk/cream, green tea OTHER: eggs, beans, legumes, olives, extra virgin olive oil, apple cider vinegar, fibre, whole grains, prebiotics, probiotics, dark chocolate, honey
Really simple meal ideas	Avocado on wholegrain toast, with sliced boiled egg and grilled tomatoes. Grilled fish, wilted spinach with a squeeze of lemon juice, wholemeal rice. Mackerel flaked over watercress salad, with grated carrot, tomatoes, sunflower seeds. Wholemeal pasta with tomatoes, peppers, spinach, olives, and garlic. Broccoli, cauliflower, mixed pepper chilli with kidney beans. Homemade kale crisps: kale roasted with salt and apple cider vinegar. Fruit dipped in melted dark chocolate. Coconut milk warmed up with turmeric and cinnamon.

Low Histamine Diet	
Condition it deals with	Excess histamine in the body and/or histamine intolerance. Histamine is a chemical that is released when the body is being attacked — it is part of the immune response and what makes us sneeze or have a runny nose if we encounter something we are allergic to. It is also helpful for digestion, blood pressure, and hormone regulation.
What the diet does	A low histamine diet reduces the amount of histamine in the body. Some foods contain histamine and some foods encourage the release of histamine in the body. This diet may be accompanied by consumption of a dietary supplement containing the diamine oxidase (DAO) enzyme, which helps to break down histamine in the body.
Why it might be relevant to us	Vaccines can trigger histamine release as part of the immune response. Some of us feel like we are having an allergic or intolerant reaction to lots of things since being vaccinated. Some of us may have had tests that indicate high levels of histamine or DAO enzyme in our bodies, or we may have tested for MCAS (mast cell activation syndrome), which is the release of an excessive amount of histamine. Some of us have symptoms that may indicate histamine intolerance, such as headaches, congestion, fatigue, or digestive problems. Some of us may have already suffered with allergies or intolerances, before vaccination. And some of us may have been advised to try taking antihistamines and found that our symptoms improved.
Foods to avoid	Anything fermented/pickled/canned/processed; mackerel, tuna, sardines; tomatoes, eggplant/aubergine, spinach, sprouts, avocado; kiwi, plums, papaya, citrus, strawberries, bananas, dried fruit; coffee, kombucha, cocoa; beans, soy, peanuts, vinegar, olives, chocolate, alcohol, leftovers (the longer food is left, the higher the histamine content).
Helpful foods	FISH: trout, cod, freshly caught, wild, unprocessed FRUIT: apples, blueberries, grapes, coconut, pineapple, non-citrus fruits, most other fresh fruit above in "Foods to avoid" VEG: broccoli, watercress, sweet potatoes, red peppers, courgettes, red cabbage, onions, most other fresh veg except above in "Foods to avoid" NUTS & SEEDS: chia seeds HERBS & SPICES: ginger, turmeric, tarragon, thyme, parsley DRINKS: plant milks, herbal teas, black tea, green tea OTHER: freshly cooked meat (not the leftovers), eggs, olive oil, rapeseed oil, coconut oil, grains
Really simple meal ideas	Baked cod with sweet potato wedges and steamed broccoli. Omelette with onions and parsley. Baked apple and blueberries with coconut cream. Watercress salad with spring onions, boiled egg, red peppers, and chia seeds. Cottage pie with sweet potato mash. Broccoli, onion, courgette soup. Courgette/zucchini noodles with red peppers, red onions, and olive oil. Baked chicken skewers with red peppers, onions, and sweet potato chunks.

Low-Mould/Mold Diet	
Condition it deals with	Mould allergies or a build-up of mycotoxins in the body — invisible poisonous substances that can colonise the human body. Historical or repeated mould exposure can damage the immune system, and cause inflammation and/or excessive histamine production. Some people are genetically predisposed to mould poisoning.
What the diet does	A Low-Mould Diet — along with the removal of any exposure to mould — limits the consumption of any foods that naturally contain mould, inhibits the continued growth of any mould within the body, and helps the body detox from any historical mould poisoning. It is also intended to improve the body's ability to absorb more nutrients.
Why it might be relevant to us	Most people have been exposed to mould at some point in their lifetime — and many of us (especially in the northern hemisphere) are exposed to it as part of our daily lives, even now. Our bodies may have been dealing with mycotoxin colonies without us even knowing it, perhaps for years, putting pressure on our immune system, creating inflammation, and causing a range of allergic-type symptoms. Some of us may have the mould gene (HLA-DR) or have tested positive for mycotoxins in our urine. Note: Possible mycotoxin exposure in mammals is a known disruptive factor in vaccination programmes conducted in animals, who do not respond as expected and instead are found to have a weakened immune system response to both the vaccine and subsequent infections.
Foods to avoid	Grains, dairy, dried fruit, mushrooms, coffee (unless it is certified mycotoxin-free), refined sugars, refined rice/flour, peanuts, mycotoxin-exposed nuts/seeds/chocolate/ spices/tea, cured meats, cheese, alcohol, anything fermented/pickled/canned, anything that has been stored/transported for a long period of time. Inflammatory foods.
Helpful foods	FISH: wild salmon FRUIT: blueberries, blackberries, raspberries, apples (low sugar fruits) VEG: kale, spinach, cauliflower, broccoli, rocket, Brussels sprouts, watercress, purple sweet potato, squash, onion, leek, garlic, parsnip NUTS & SEEDS: fridge-stored almonds or walnuts HERBS & SPICES: thyme, coriander, basil, oregano, ginger, cinnamon, turmeric DRINKS: mycotoxin-free coffee, green tea, coconut milk OTHER: eggs, grass-fed meat (because animal feed is known to contain mycotoxins), olive oil, any coconut products (it's an anti-fungal), raw honey, anything to support the liver while detoxing.
Really simple meal ideas	Grilled salmon with steamed veg. Salmon soup with mixed veg, coconut cream, fresh coriander, and chilli. Lamb with vegetables roasted in coconut oil and thyme. Chicken with mashed sweet potato and squash. Omelette with spinach, onion, and oregano. Watercress salad with roasted cauliflower, toasted almonds, basil, and olive oil. Berries and apples cooked with coconut cream and cinnamon. Leek and sweet potato soup.

Small Intestinal Bacterial Overgrowth (SIBO) Diet	
Condition it deals with	Our small intestine contains microbes (bacteria and fungus) that help us digest food, absorb nutrients, and build a strong immune system. SIBO is a condition where unhelpful bacteria increase and affect our ability to digest food properly, resulting in long-term physical, cognitive, and psychological difficulties as well as stomach problems.
What the diet does	The SIBO diet involves eliminating foods that the unhelpful bacteria love, and generally involves eating low-FODMAP foods. In very simple terms, this means avoiding foods that ferment. The diet effectively starves the unhelpful bacteria, which gradually leave the body. The diet can incorporate the use of certain antibiotics to speed up the process.
Why it might be relevant to us	Some of us may have been living with gastrointestinal problems for years before the vaccine. Some of us may have had to deal with them soon after vaccination — perhaps our immune system couldn't cope with both the vaccine and any unhelpful bacteria. Some of us may even have found ourselves dealing with gastrointestinal problems months after starting to follow an improved diet designed to help with our vaccine symptoms, especially if that diet contained lots of fruit and vegetables. Bad bacteria love all that healthy food we've been eating and don't have much incentive to leave our gut if that's what we're giving them. The SIBO diet might also be relevant to us because of the key role that healthy bacteria play in supporting our recovery from the adverse reaction.
Foods to avoid	Natural or added sugars, honey, sweeteners, anything containing gum, added fibre, beans, potatoes, probiotics, prebiotics, starch powders, canned vegetables, seaweeds, chia seeds, seed flour, soy, onions, garlic (whole or powdered), balsamic vinegar, whole wheat products, multigrain products, high-sugar fruits such as apples.
Helpful foods	FISH: any FRUIT: blueberries, strawberries, raspberries, citrus, grapes, kiwi, papaya, pineapple, ginger, rhubarb VEG: peppers, tomatoes, cucumber, eggplant/aubergine, carrots, squash, broccoli, pumpkin, leafy greens (especially rocket, kale) NUTS & SEEDS: keep to a minimum HERBS & SPICES: oregano, ginger DRINKS: chamomile tea, hibiscus tea, green tea, mint tea OTHER: Meat, organ meats, eggs, olive oil, coconut oil, olives, dark chocolate, unsweetened protein powders
Really simple meal ideas	Rocket salad with peppers, tomatoes, cucumber, olives, olive oil, lemon juice. Mixed berry bowl with nuts and gum-free coconut cream. Omelette with red peppers, tomatoes, black olives, oregano, cayenne pepper. Chicken liver pate on gluten-free crackers. Coconut flour muffins (add blueberries/dark chocolate/cacao). Protein powder shakes with any fruit and unsweetened non-dairy milk. Carrot and fresh coriander soup. Baked fish/meat with lemon/oregano and steamed vegetables.

Anticoagulation/Endothelial Repair Diet	
Condition it deals with	This deals with two conditions: One: "sticky" blood (blood that has an increased tendency to clot), and can include microclotting. Two: blood vessel dysfunction, which can be caused by damage to the lining of the vessels or a tendency for the vessels to narrow. Also known as microvascular disease.
What the diet does	Unlike the diet plans in previous pages, this is not a "known regime," as such, but rather a plan that helps deal with these two conditions. It incorporates food that keeps the blood thin and flowing smoothly, and also promotes cellular repair of the blood vessels, and requires very careful monitoring if you are on any blood-thinning medication.
Why it might be relevant to us	Some of us are struggling with having blood drawn, find ourselves bruising easily and inexplicably, and have symptoms that seem to indicate a change in our blood vessels, such as bulging or brightly coloured veins. Some of us have accidentally discovered that we seem to feel much better after we have had a number of blood tests or having tried therapeutic phlebotomy. Some of us have found relief with forms of blood dialysis, whereby the blood is cleaned before being returned to the body. It is now well-documented that people suffering with Long Covid seem to be dealing with a microclotting problem, and many of our symptoms seem to match those of Long Covid sufferers. It would not be surprising to find that we are also dealing with coagulation and endothelial problems.
Foods to avoid	Anything containing Vitamin K: asparagus, broccoli, sprouts, cauliflower, green onions, leafy greens (kale, parsley, spinach) BUT leafy greens have so many other benefits that garlic may be consumed to counteract the negative impact. Avoid anything that triggers inflammation.
Helpful foods	FISH: salmon, tuna, trout FRUIT: purple grapes, raspberries, strawberries, blueberries, pineapple, watermelon, citrus, banana, mango, avocado VEG: seaweed, beetroot, garlic, carrots, cucumber, pumpkin, red peppers NUTS & SEEDS: sunflower seeds, pumpkin seeds, almonds, peanuts HERBS & SPICES: turmeric, cinnamon, ginger, cayenne DRINKS: chamomile tea, pomegranate juice, red wine OTHER: beef, chicken, pork, organ meats, virgin olive oil, dark chocolate, peanut butter, foods that contain nitrates (they open up blood vessels) such as leafy greens but see above for contradictory effect
Really simple meal ideas	Avocado and poached egg on seeded bread. Mixed fruit bowl with nuts and seeds, coconut cream and cinnamon. Shot of pomegranate juice and half a squeezed lemon, with hot water. Beetroot, carrot, ginger juice or smoothie. Miso soup with salmon, seaweed, and garlic. Berries dipped in melted dark chocolate and peanut butter. Chicken liver pate with garlic on seeded bread. Roasted meat with beetroot, carrot, garlic, and oregano, served with steamed kale.

Your Gut Health

Whatever level of approach you decide to try, at some point you might find that the subject of gut health comes up. Gut health refers to the state of your entire digestive system, starting with your attitude toward food, including how your brain processes information about food, and the food's entire physical journey from your mouth to your anus. It is a *huge* topic, and you'll find almost three billion results if you enter the phrase "gut health" into Google. There are thousands of books written about it, countless online seminars available on it, and plenty of highly educated professionals who have dedicated their lives to helping people deal with a myriad of health problems by addressing their gut health. You really do have enough on your plate right now (no pun intended), but this is an area that you probably can't ignore if you want to get the most out of whatever food programme you're going to incorporate into your ongoing recovery. Here are just a few basics to start with:

- **Food preparation:** Take your time in preparing your meals, think about the benefits they will bring, and create positive associations with the entire process.
- **Chewing:** Chew every mouthful really slowly, and chew until the food is no longer solid. Take your time over the meal. Focus on it (try not to watch TV while eating).
- **Digestion:** Take your time in getting up after your meal. Let it settle into your body comfortably. Don't rush on to the next activity you may have planned. Don't "eat on the go."
- **Eat probiotics and prebiotics:** Incorporate foods that will put and feed healthy bacteria in your gut (this obviously depends on whether your food programme allows it or not).
- **Reduce inflammation:** See Anti-Inflammatory Diet.
- **Avoid antibiotics:** Antibiotics interfere with the bacteria present in the gut, so if you do take them then the gut bacteria may need to be rebalanced.
- **Consume bone broth:** Along with numerous other benefits, bone broth is believed to repair intestinal lining.
- **Have a good poo:** Take your time. Don't hold it in, and don't rush it out.

If all we do is start *really* taking our time with every stage in our digestive process, then that alone will contribute toward improved gut health.

Combining Approaches

You might find that several approaches resonate with you, so you will want to create your own diet as part of your recovery plan. I wanted to reduce inflammation, but I had also been exposed to mould. I had some signs of SIBO in the years prior to vaccination but was showing strong signs of clotting problems post-vaccination. I started off with a diet that boosted my immune system but ended up adding elements of every single diet I summarised on the previous pages.

Trying to deal with possible contributing factors to health issues that are either caused, triggered, or exacerbated by the vaccine can be incredibly overwhelming. You might start off by increasing the amount of fruit and vegetables you eat, only to find that this is feeding SIBO that you didn't even know you had, so then you have that to deal with on top of everything else. Here are a few ways you can simplify things if you find yourself dealing with multiple issues:

- **One month at a time:** Spend a whole month focused on just one thing, whether it is Level One where you're trying to avoid anything that makes you feel worse, or whether you want to be more specific and follow one of the programmes I've summarised.
- **Slowly add new elements:** If you feel that your food plan is working for you but there might be other things you need to address, incorporate the new things rather than switching to a completely new programme. For example, you might be eating nuts to boost your immune system, but then suspect you might be dealing with mould, so you decide to cut out peanuts (or even all nuts) for a month and monitor how you feel.
- **Prioritise:** Decide which condition is most important to you and follow the plan for that one, perhaps with a few elements of other plans added but not quite as strictly. For example, at the time of writing, anticoagulation/endothelial repair is my absolute priority, so I strictly follow that plan, but I'm still keeping up with an anti-SIBO diet, while incorporating elements of the low-mould diet.
- **Give food items a score:** Dealing with three possible contributing factors? Perhaps you suspect you're dealing with low histamine but also SIBO and clotting problems? You could give a food item a maximum score of 3, depending on whether it meets the criteria for all three health conditions. Then design your own plan based only on foods that score a 2 or a 3.

Creating Your Own Diet
This chart can be used to keep track of foods that you think will help (or hinder) a combination of possible contributing factors, as well as take into account any food allergies or intolerances you may have had before vaccination.

My Personal Recovery Diet	
Possible contributing factors I want to address (number in order of priority)	Anti-Inflammatory / Low-Histamine / Mould / SIBO / Blood & Vascular
Other pre-existing food-related issues to be aware of (e.g., allergies/ intolerances/surgeries)	
Foods to avoid	
Helpful foods (include drinks, herbs, spices)	
Really simple meal ideas	

Modifying Your Existing Diet

Use this chart to keep track of some simple ways you can change your favourite meals so that they incorporate elements of your new food plan. I've given you a few examples that I've used.

Meal	Modification
Poached egg on toast	Use whole grain bread, spread avocado on first, grill some tomatoes with oregano sprinkled on them.
Omelette	Use coconut oil instead of butter, courgettes and peppers instead of ham and cheese, and add oregano and cayenne pepper.
Soups	Use bone broth instead of stock, add fresh herbs instead of processed flavouring, use fresh tomatoes instead of tinned.
	Add your own ideas below.

Shopping Lists

Caroline's food shopping list

watercress
spinach
kale
courgettes
red peppers
broccoli
beetroot
avocado
tomatoes
blueberries
strawberries
raspberries
purple grapes
pineapple
papaya
watermelon
lemons
sunflower seeds
pumpkin seeds
seed bread
olives
olive oil
salmon
mackerel
lamb bones
dark chocolate
cacao powder
hemp powder
coconut milk
coconut cream (no gum)
pomegranate juice
green tea
hibiscus tea
mycotoxin-free coffee
turmeric
ginger
cayenne
cinnamon
oregano
seaweed snack

My food shopping list

(take your time to add your staple foods here so you can easily hand this to someone, send it as a photo, or take it shopping yourself)

My food shopping list
(spare — you can rip this page out)

My food shopping list
(spare — you can rip this page out)

Caroline's 15-Minute Meals

I post a lot of pictures on my social media of the meals that I eat, and people are always asking me for my recipes. I rarely follow any, but here are some of my favourite go-to meals that meet my particular food criteria, are super easy to make, really tasty, and take less than fifteen minutes to put together.

Spanish-Inspired Breakfast Omelette with Fruit Bowl

Ingredients (per person):

> 1 tbsp. coconut oil
> 1/4 red pepper, chopped
> handful black olives, halved, in olive oil
> 1/4 courgette, chopped
> handful spinach
> 2 cherry tomatoes, quartered
> 2 free-range eggs
> 1 tsp. dried oregano
> 1/2 tsp. SCT chorizo panko (or 1/4 tsp. cayenne)
> juice of half a lemon
> handful fresh basil leaves

Method:

1. Melt the coconut oil in a small frying pan.
2. Add red pepper, olives, and courgette to frying pan. Fry for a few minutes, stirring occasionally.
3. Add spinach and tomato to frying pan. Stir.
4. Break eggs into a bowl and add oregano and panko/cayenne, then mix with a fork.
5. Give the veg a final stir before pouring egg-mix on, then turn the grill on high ready for puffing up the omelette.
6. Leave the egg/veg mix to cook while chopping fruit to ensure this meal means you will be "eating the rainbow" (I usually choose papaya and blueberries).
7. Put the frying pan under the grill and, when the omelette has puffed up, put it on a plate, squeeze half a lemon over it, and garnish with the fresh basil.

This meal is anti-inflammatory, anti-mould, anti-SIBO, and supports blood and vascular health.

Caroline's 15-Minute Meals

Super Dooper Porridge

Ingredients (per person):

> 50g gluten-free porridge
> 250ml coconut milk
> handful mixed berries
> 1/3 banana, chopped
> 1 tsp. cinnamon
> 1 tsp. hemp protein powder

Method:

1. Put all ingredients in a pan, mix thoroughly, bring to the boil, simmer for 5 minutes.

This meal is anti-inflammatory, and supports blood and vascular health.

Rainbow Salad & Black Coffee with Cinnamon

Ingredients (per person):

> 2 cherry tomatoes, quartered
> 1/4 carrot, grated
> handful watercress or rocket (arugula) leaves
> 6 cubes cooked beetroot
> boiled egg, quartered
> pumpkin seeds
> drizzle olive oil
> juice of half a lemon
> mycotoxin-free coffee
> 1/8 tsp. cinnamon

Method:

2. Put vegetables, egg, and pumpkin seeds in a bowl.
3. Drizzle with olive oil and lemon juice.
4. Add the cinnamon to the coffee.

This meal is anti-inflammatory, anti-mould, anti-SIBO, and supports blood and vascular health.

Caroline's 15-Minute Meals

Thai-Inspired Salmon Soup

Ingredients (per person):

        boneless, wild salmon steak

        500ml bone broth

        1/2 tsp. cayenne pepper

        1/2 tsp. curry powder

        2 handfuls any mixed veg. (broccoli is lovely in this)

        handful fresh coriander leaves

        100ml coconut cream (no added gum)

Method:

1. Put salmon steak in pan, cover with bone broth, bring up to the boil. Keep boiling throughout next stages.
2. Add cayenne and curry powders.
3. Add mixed veg.
4. Add coriander leaves.
5. Take off the heat and stir in coconut cream before serving.

This meal is anti-inflammatory, anti-mould, anti-SIBO, low-histamine, and supports blood, vascular, and gut health.

Caroline's favourite drinks

    Pomegranate juice, juice of half a lemon, hot water.

    Organic green tea.

    Mycotoxin-free black coffee.

    Organic hibiscus/peppermint/chamomile tea.

    Coconut milk with tsp. each of cinnamon and turmeric.

Caroline's favourite snacks

    Stick of celery, carrot, or banana covered in almond butter.

    Boiled egg.

    Handful pumpkin/sunflower seeds.

    Half an avocado.

    Kale baked in the oven with olive oil and Himalayan salt.

Dietary Supplements

Dietary supplements is another area where there are countless websites, online videos, and professionals; not to mention there are so many different opinions about dietary supplements that it is difficult to know who to trust. It's easy to get overwhelmed and start worrying about what you could, should, or shouldn't be adding to your diet, and that's before you even start thinking about the cost.

If you want to give your diet a boost then you should easily be able to find lists of a few things you can supplement with by searching online, for example, for "anti-inflammatory supplements," etc. Basic supplements can be found in your local supermarket, another level up can be found in health food shops or pharmacies, and, if you really want to go for the maximum quality you can get, then there are online pharmacies that specifically supply very high-quality supplements.

The chart below and overleaf will help you keep track of which supplements might benefit you, depending on what might be showing up in any test results, or which specific food plan you're following. For example, I had a less-than-optimal result in a Vitamin D test — Vitamin D plays a role in the immune system but is tricky to get from diet alone, and I live in the UK where we don't have sunlight all year round — so I supplement. I'm prioritising my blood so I also take an anticoagulant, but I'm also trying to detox from mould so I take something to support my liver. Lots to manage, and hopefully this will help you manage yours ...

Supplement name	Why it might help me	How and when to take	Brand	Where to get it

Dietary Supplements (cont.)

Supplement name	Why it might help me	How and when to take	Brand	Where to get it

Food "Hacks"

Making changes to our food habits can seem really overwhelming, especially at a time when we're already overwhelmed. Here are a few ways to simplify the process, and they can be implemented regardless of which level or which programme you've decided to follow.

- **Get a slow cooker:** This will save you so much time, and it won't matter *at all* if you forget whether you've got something cooking or not. You can literally throw whatever you like in and just leave it, and it's perfect for making bone broth. If people ask you whether they can help you at all, or if you need anything, ask them for a slow cooker.

- **Get a blender:** When you really can't cook anything, you can throw in a load of fruit, some protein powder, and some non-dairy milk, and whizz it all up in minutes. Again, if someone wants to help, ask for a blender.

- **Abandon recipes:** If you're at the stage where following a recipe is challenging, then don't follow one. Stick with some basics until your cognitive functions are a little better: grilled meat or fish, steamed veg, soups where you just put whatever you want in a pot, salads. Add some herbs or spices to start with and just add more as you go along. Don't let the stress of following a recipe spoil what should be an enjoyable and healing process for you.

- **Make a go-to shopping list:** Make one shopping list that can be used for every shopping trip. Whether you shop online or in person, or someone else does your food shopping, this will save so much time, energy, and possibly frustration. Go back a few pages to find a list of things I always make sure are in my cupboards. There is some space there for you to make your own list when you have the inclination or capability. I've designed it so that you can rip out the whole page if you like, and it won't affect your ability to read anything else. And if someone offers to help you, your list is ready to go.

- **Modify your favourite meals:** If you're not up to trying any new meal ideas yet, then just think about how you can modify your existing favourite meals to accommodate your new food plan. It can be something as simple as adding oregano for anticoagulation.

On the page before my shopping list, I've included some ideas that I use, with space for you to put your own.

- **Eating out:** Assuming you have the energy to even contemplate eating out (which I know I didn't for *months*), it might be an idea to think ahead and check the menu, which many places put online now. While there might not be many items that meet your new food criteria, most places will have a meat/fish with vegetables option, or a fairly decent salad, and those will satisfy most of the food plans featured here. I double check whether they're using butter and ask if they can use olive oil instead, and I ask for half a lemon instead of dressing.
- **Snacking on the go:** If you know you'll be out and about and will need something quick to keep you going, then put a little snack box together that contains your safe foods. My snack box usually includes a boiled egg, celery with almond butter, and some pumpkin seeds, grapes, and dark chocolate.

Autophagy

An entirely different approach to diet as part of a recovery programme might involve fasting to induce autophagy. "Auto" "phagy" literally means "self" "eating," and it involves getting the body into a state whereby it is not consuming nutrients from food, but instead is breaking down damaged cellular components and removing them from the body — a kind of "house cleaning" process that also helps restore cellular health when done on a periodic (not daily) basis. This technique is used by some people as a way of trying to prevent some cancers, neurodegenerative diseases, and diabetes, and Tom Bunker is known among the Long Covid and vaccine-injured Facebook communities as an innovative source of information on autophagy as a way of dealing with our symptoms.

Professional Diet Support

While doctors are usually able to provide basic advice on nutrition support, it is rare to find one who can provide specific advice regarding targetted nutrition or nutrition for the purpose of recovery from anything, let alone from a vaccine. For this you will need the expert advice of a nutritionist, or a Functional Medicine practitioner, although some holistic practitioners such as acupuncturists and homeopaths also have knowledge about the healing benefits of specific diets. More information about professionals available to support us is in Chapter 5.

Ending Diet Restrictions

None of the diet plans we might be considering are designed to be long-term, permanent diets, and in fact some of them (such as SIBO) are specifically designed to be short-term, and only followed for a matter of months. At some point we'll probably want to add foods to our diet that we have chosen to temporarily not eat, and, along with some excitement, there can also be a certain amount of anxiety regarding adding foods back into our diet that we haven't consumed for a while, especially if we're starting to see improvements in our symptoms.

This is where it's really important to change how we see "a setback," and instead see it as a learning opportunity: a way to learn something else about our food sensitivities or about how far along we are with our healing. I'll give you a few examples of my own.

- **Ice cream:** I went to the beach around month two. I'd been dairy-free for a month without fully understanding why, and treated myself to a clotted cream ice cream. Within an hour my stomach felt bloated and I became extremely uncomfortable. Twenty-four hours later I started hallucinating. That taught me that dairy was not helping me with recovery.
- **Cauliflower:** Around month five and fully embracing the fruit and vegetables, I made an amazing dish with cauliflower romanesco. Within an hour my stomach started swelling and making the loudest noises, and that night I was awake at 2am with what I now refer to as "EBS" (Exploding Bumhole Syndrome). The EBS continued several times a day for two weeks, and led me to learn about SIBO.
- **Gum:** My month-seven anniversary was also my fiftieth birthday. By then I'd learned to be very careful with my diet, so I made my own birthday cake with safe ingredients. I had a bit of cake for three consecutive days, as well as some gluten-free gravy both at the birthday lunch and at home on the consecutive days. On the fourth day I had a migraine, so checked the ingredients of both the cake and the gravy, and found they had xanthan gum in common, something I'd never even heard of let alone knew could cause problems.

The next page is designed for you to keep track of food items that you might be testing out as you move away from restrictive diets and toward a new stage of healing.

Food item to test	My body's response within 24 hours	Add to diet?

My Food Diary

Use this chart to keep track of how your nutrition progresses over time. You don't need to write much, and you don't need to do it every day. It takes time to develop new habits. Maybe just take a moment each week to jot down a sentence or two about what's going on with your food. It will be a great way to look back later and see how far you've come! There are other diary tools at the back of the book.

Date	What's going on with my food?

My Food Obstacles

Most of us tend to be *really* good at creating excuses for not eating well, or at telling ourselves that there are all sorts of obstacles that get in the way of us grabbing food that might not be the healthiest for us. We can't use those excuses or obstacles now — our health has become too important to us. We need to look for solutions, so let's get those excuses out of the way.

What is stopping me from eating in a way that helps me with recovery?	How can I remove these obstacles?

We Are All Different

Food can be a complicated issue for some of us. Some of us may have physical or emotional issues that turn something that could help with our recovery into something that causes us even more anxiety. Some of us do not have friends or family nearby that can help with shopping or cooking when we are at the stage or experiencing days where such things feel utterly impossible to accomplish. Some of us do not have the financial resources required to buy the best quality food, to buy from the local markets, to get hold of the most powerful supplements, or to access the best professionals working in the field of nutrition. Food can feel like a huge, overwhelming part of our recovery plan, where eating the wrong thing can make us feel dramatically worse.

Unlike the first chapter on Sleep, where all you really need to do is get as much of it as possible, as often as possible, and you *will* see an improvement in your symptoms, food isn't like that. Unfortunately, there is no "one diet fixes all" for us.

But I do believe that if we just take it one step at a time with our food, focus on the healing potential of everything that we choose to put into our bodies, and create positive associations around what may be a new way of eating, then we will not only be giving our bodies the best chance we possibly can for healing, but also be developing new habits that we can take with us into the healthy life that is waiting for us further down the recovery road.

Wheel of Healing Update

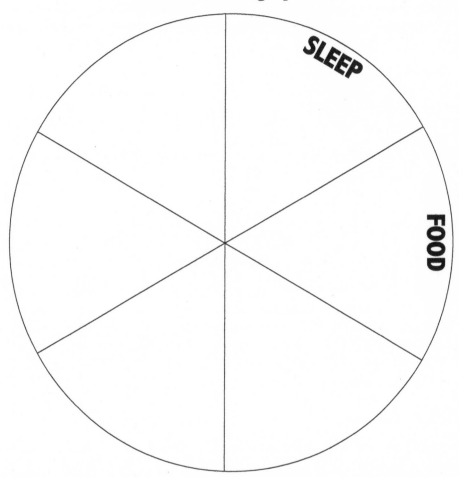

Before you add some notes about your nutrition plan, first take a moment to update your Sleep actions. Ask yourself whether your sleep has improved. Does it need a bit more effort or have you managed to achieve a sleep pattern that is maximising your recovery?

Then in the Food section, make some notes on what approach you'd like to try with your food. What do you feel you need to eat more or less of? Is there a nutrition programme that you want to try at this stage of your recovery? Any supplements you'd like to add? Try to keep your notes simple here. It is intended to be an overview of your healing plan.

My Food Resources (books/websites/articles/recipes)

Other Notes/Thoughts on Food

Before you start this chapter ...

Take a moment to note your *feelings* about your symptoms — not the symptoms themselves because that can be quite overwhelming. There are activities in this chapter to help you think about the symptoms in a way that is intended to help you feel less overwhelmed. So first, just make some notes on how you feel about all these things happening to your body right now. Take some time to put those feelings into words. Don't rush, and know that it's totally understandable if this makes you upset.

CHAPTER 3: SYMPTOMS

SUMMARY

Create a visual representation of your symptoms.
Tackle one symptom at a time rather than all of them.
Symptom flares can be tools that help us learn more about our health.
Full-body healing techniques can be helpful for ongoing recovery.
Focusing excessively on a symptom's cause may distract from healing.

Our symptoms seem to be never-ending. It feels like one thing after another, more often than not with multiple symptoms happening at the same time. Once we think we've got one of them under control, then another one flares up and makes life unmanageable again. Lack of sleep, or the "wrong" kind of food, can make all the difference as to whether we have a half-decent day or an absolutely terrible one. Keeping track of all the symptoms feels like a full-time job, for which you've had no training whatsoever. It's not just all the weird symptoms that are overwhelming — it's the management of those symptoms too.

On the following pages are some exercises that can help you keep track of your symptoms, help you keep focused on the one/s you want to prioritise, and note ways of possibly dealing with the symptoms. The examples I've used relate to my own symptoms, and any notes on what worked for me doesn't imply that the solution I found will necessarily work for you — we are all different.

First, there is a diagram in which you can note all of your own symptoms. This will be helpful in putting them all in one place, is designed to be easy to add to (or cross out) as you go along, and is a simple way of showing anybody else (medical or otherwise) what exactly you're dealing with.

Symptom Record
(using Caroline's symptoms as an example)

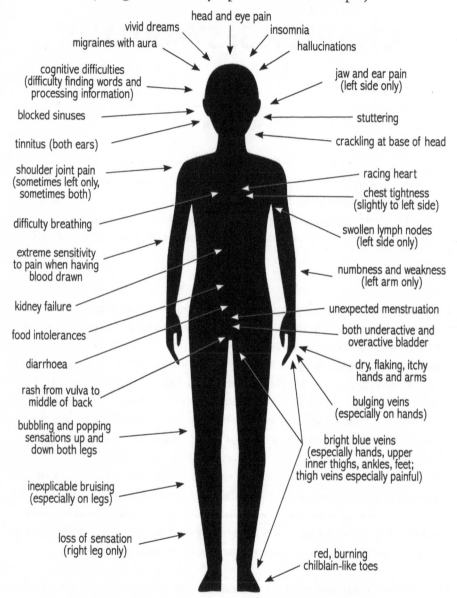

vivid dreams

head and eye pain

insomnia

migraines with aura

hallucinations

cognitive difficulties
(difficulty finding words and
processing information)

jaw and ear pain
(left side only)

blocked sinuses

stuttering

tinnitus (both ears)

crackling at base of head

shoulder joint pain
(sometimes left only,
sometimes both)

racing heart

chest tightness
(slightly to left side)

difficulty breathing

swollen lymph nodes
(left side only)

extreme sensitivity
to pain when having
blood drawn

numbness and weakness
(left arm only)

kidney failure

unexpected menstruation

food intolerances

both underactive and
overactive bladder

diarrhoea

dry, flaking, itchy
hands and arms

rash from vulva to
middle of back

bulging veins
(especially on hands)

bubbling and popping
sensations up and
down both legs

bright blue veins
(especially hands, upper
inner thighs, ankles, feet;
thigh veins especially painful)

inexplicable bruising
(especially on legs)

loss of sensation
(right leg only)

red, burning
chilblain-like toes

other: fatigue, excessive sleeping/yawning/crying, internal vibrations,
suicidal thoughts, agoraphobia, random shooting pains, hypercoagulation

54

Creating Your Own Symptom Record

If you plan on using your own Symptom Record for the purpose of showing others your symptoms from the start, then note everything you can remember. This might be useful for anyone who is providing you with healthcare support and wants to know the full picture of what you have been dealing with.

You can add more details, such as date of symptom onset, or length of time the symptom is/was present. You could colour code symptoms if you're already seeing patterns in your symptoms; for example, anything indicating gastrointestinal issues could be one colour, and anything neurological could be another; but I like to know what patterns others see so I don't colour code mine. I prefer to keep the record simple. Just looking at the symptoms alone is enough to deal with!

Using Your Symptom Record

Apart from being able to easily show someone your symptoms, your Symptom Record will help you identify which symptom you want to make a priority, and therefore help prevent that overwhelming feeling that is so common among us. By focusing on one symptom at a time, we can take steps to deal with that symptom from a position of strength, empowerment, and control, rather than that panic-laden game of medical "Whack-a-mole" that we can easily get drawn into.

The most debilitating symptom for me in the early weeks was the constant head and eye pain — it was relentless. So when I felt able to be a bit more proactive in my recovery, I made that a priority, and experimented with all sorts of ways to make the pain go away, as well as live with it while it was happening. I think I finally started seeing some relief at about day 42, and during those six weeks there were a couple of other symptoms that I started to tackle as well, but only when I felt up to it. After you've created your own Symptom Record, there are some pages for you to make notes on how you might try to deal with your symptoms, with some examples from my own experience to give you ideas.

One of the best uses of a Symptom Record like this is that it can be a wonderfully encouraging record of how far you have come! When a symptom is no longer present for you, you can either cross it out or highlight it, but not erase it, so that you can still see it. Now it shows something you have overcome or at least learned to manage so that it is no longer a problem for you.

My Symptom Record

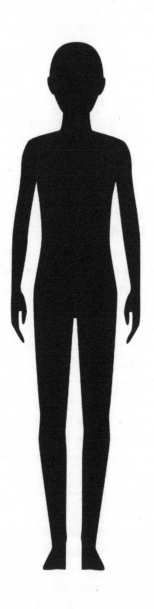

My Symptom Record (spare)

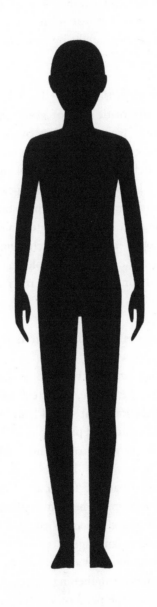

Symptom Management

Once you've noted all of your symptoms on the diagram, try to tackle them just one at a time. Either start with the one that is bothering you the most, or the one that feels the most manageable, then think of ways you might be able to deal with that. You can then focus your research on to dealing with that one specific symptom, and try to avoid getting caught up in dealing with *all* your symptoms in one go.

If I think about my own symptoms, the one that bothered me the most at first was the cognitive disability, so I made a list of everything that I could draw upon to get my brain to work again. This included lots of sleep, food for my brain, and the removal of anything that could tax my brain in any way. When the head and eye pain became the most debilitating symptom, then I switched my approach to still maintain the habits I had developed to support my brain's recovery, but made the head and eye pain my priority and learned some techniques to deal with pain. When diarrhoea became the most debilitating, then that became my focus. In doing all of that, I developed my own, ever-changing way of dealing with my worst symptoms, tackling just one at a time. Employing that methodical approach kept me from feeling overwhelmed, and helped me feel that I was in charge of my own recovery.

Whatever symptom/s we are dealing with, we can draw upon the same methods to help alleviate them:

- **Nutrition:** Our diets can be tweaked to specifically deal with certain symptoms; for example, when excessive clotting became my priority, I added foods that would help keep my blood thin, such as pomegranate juice and pineapple.
- **Brain rewiring:** We can help our brains "relearn" abilities that have become difficult for us by doing certain exercises that stimulate the affected part of the brain. This applies to many different skills. For example, when my mathematical skills evaded me, I did lots of Sudoku; when I struggled with word recall, I started learning another language.
- **Physiotherapy:** For physical challenges, especially those affecting our limbs, very gentle strengthening exercises can help, and can often be done without the need of a professional. For example,

when my left arm and shoulder became weak and frequently numb, I used only the left side of my body when doing things that I would ordinarily have done with my right, such as brushing my teeth.

- **Stimulation:** Stimulating parts of the body that are symptomatic can also help promote blood flow to the area. This can be achieved through simple self-massage (obviously, only if you can reach the area!) and also through employing healing therapies, such as acupuncture, that are specifically intended to stimulate the body's own healing response.

Use the pages overleaf to make notes on your symptoms and different things you can try in order to alleviate them. I don't recommend filling out the boxes all in one go — just focus on one thing at a time. If you manage to alleviate one symptom in a matter of days, then by all means go on to the next one, but I would recommend spending one month dealing with just one symptom. Allow the healing strategies you employ to tackle that one symptom to become part of your daily routine, and give yourself time for your body to respond to your efforts.

Caroline's Examples of Symptom Management

Symptom	Healing Solutions to try	Results/notes
Ear and jaw pain	• garlic oil drops • massage jaw joint • acupuncture • anti-inflammatory food	Drops and massage effective within days. Had acupuncture to promote further healing.
Blocked sinuses	• sinus massage • Himalayan salt pipe inhaler • anti-histamine tablets • low histamine foods	Sinuses fully cleared within two weeks. Continued with low histamine diet.
Crackling at base of head	• cold shower aimed at back of neck • craniosacral massage • acupuncture	Disappeared after a couple of months. Suspect the cold shower most effective.
Extreme sensitivity to pain while having blood drawn	• extra hydration 24 hours before draws • hot bath one hour before blood draws • breathing techniques for pain • positive visual associations during draws	Difficult to say which one is most effective. Continue combining all.

My Ongoing Symptom Management

Symptom	Healing Solutions to try	Results/notes

My Ongoing Symptom Management

Symptom	Healing Solutions to try	Results/notes

Symptom "Flares"

Many of us who have been dealing with all this for more than six months have probably already experienced a "flare." This is when, despite what you think are your best efforts, one symptom (or more) suddenly seems to get much worse, and you're not sure why. It's confusing and disheartening, especially if you're putting a lot of effort into your recovery. I think it took three incidents of "flaring" for me to completely change my attitude toward it. I stopped feeling angry and frustrated, and instead started looking at each incident as an opportunity to learn something new about my body and what it needed in order to recover. I turned something that actually distressed me quite a bit into something helpful and empowering.

The chart on the next page should help you keep track of your own flares, identify what might have been behind them, and make any necessary changes to your recovery plan. The following chart contains a few of my own examples.

Flare	Anything different going on with ...			What I learned
	my sleep?	my food?	anything else?	
Hallucination, migraine, knife-like head pain	N/A	Ate ice cream after being dairy-free for 1 month.	N/A	Continue dairy-free. Test again later but be prepared for consequences!
Severe joint pain in both shoulders	N/A	N/A	Caught a cold	Be prepared for other (normal) health conditions to reactivate symptoms.
Fatigue	N/A	N/A	Two consecutive 8-hr days working.	Try working alternate days.
Cognitive functions not working	Neighbour kept me awake.	N/A	N/A	Talk to neighbour, get earplugs, try melatonin on noisy nights.

Sometimes, despite all our best efforts to heal, these flares can seemingly come out of nowhere. We might try our best to understand what triggered them, but find ourselves completely baffled. At that point, I try to stop, take a breather from managing my health, and just go with the flare. Stop fighting. Find the patience to wait for it to pass. And it always does.

My Symptom Flares

Flare	Anything different going on with ...			What I learned
	my sleep?	my food?	anything else?	

Full-Body Healing

Most people working in non-pharmaceutical areas of healthcare would probably advocate full-body healing over symptom-specific healing: the exact opposite of what I've just explained in this chapter so far. But for a number of reasons, I stand by my suggestions of focusing on healing one symptom at a time.

First, when you're in the middle of dealing with such a large number of overwhelming symptoms, the idea of tackling them using more holistic, full-body methods seems a bit like putting out a fire using drops of water. It *feels* like you'll never get anywhere, that it will be a never-ending battle, and all the while there could be even more damage raging on and on. This is not encouraging at all. Whereas if you break down your struggles and tackle one symptom at a time, focusing on each one, then you're more likely to be aware of any improvement.

Second, when you're looking at full-body healing, it can be very easy to spend hours and hours researching all sorts of non-specific health conditions that *sound* a bit like yours but then again don't really, and you end up feeling overwhelmed, helpless, and hopeless. Whereas if you focus *only* on finding possible healing solutions for a very specific symptom, then you'll find a few ideas fairly quickly, and be able to stay focused on them for a month (or however long you feel you need to prioritise that symptom), and you'll be more aware of improvements. I find it to be a much more empowering way of managing recovery.

Third, being able to cross off each of those symptoms as you progress is going to make you feel awesome. I didn't actually realise until I wrote this chapter that I've had around forty different symptoms to deal with. Now, eleven months in, I'm dealing with twelve symptoms. They're pretty big symptoms that greatly affect my life on a daily basis, *but*, purely from a numbers perspective, twelve is a huge improvement on forty. I might still have a long way to go — I might not even get much further than this — but I have quantifiable evidence of how far I've come.

While I do advocate dealing with one symptom at a time rather than trying to "fix" everything at once, full-body healing techniques can be helpful in giving your body extra support in general as you recover. If you're making sleep a priority, and eating in a way that maximises your body's chance of recovering in general, then you are already supporting full-body healing.

There are a few full-body healing techniques we can easily incorporate at whatever level we feel able to (and at whatever financial cost we are able to bear). Some may seem really obvious, but they are easy to forget about when we're overwhelmed with so many symptoms to deal with. For example:

- **Breathing:** It's such a simple thing, but it's something we neglect. Taking the time to breathe deeply and slowly helps to bring about so many physical and psychological benefits. There are plenty of resources available to teach us how to breathe *properly*, and we can easily incorporate this into our recovery plan.
- **Nature:** Spending time in the *green* outdoors, whether that's in a field, a park, a forest, or just your back garden, has got to be better for us than sitting indoors.
- **Water:** Water can help us heal in many ways. This could mean spending time by the sea or a lake, going swimming if you feel able, or switching your shower to cold on the back of your neck for the last few minutes (my personal favourite).
- **Moving our bodies:** Note that I don't refer to this as "exercise." Exercise, as we knew it before the vaccine, can easily trigger flares, as many of us have found out. Simply finding ways to move our bodies, at whatever level we feel able, will help us with our healing.
- **Touch:** Hugs, massages, the stroking of a pet — all of these things are well-known to lower heart rates, help us feel calm, and promote healing.
- **Positive thoughts:** Positive thoughts *alone* are absolutely not going to get us through this, despite whatever some may say (I doubt they ever had to deal with an adverse reaction to a vaccine). But positive thinking will help with healing. Whether it's making a concerted effort to regularly experience something "joyful," or celebrating the little wins we have on our healing journey, finding ways to nurture our own positive attitude is really important.

Many professionals have dedicated their lives to working in or sharing information on a wide range of full-body healing strategies. I've included overviews of some healing practitioners in a later chapter on Consultants, which may provide you with further ideas on how to support your full-body healing efforts. Practitioners with a holistic approach can be invaluable as we deal with such a wide range of complicated symptoms that affect our whole body.

These pages are spaces for you to keep track of any full-body healing techniques that you explore, and how you feel they are working for you. This might help you then identify what you'd like to include in your ongoing recovery plan, and the frequency with which you'd like to include it. I've included a few of my own to start you off.

My Full-Body Healing Strategies

Strategy	How it works for me	Frequency	Resources/notes
Deep breathing	Increases oxygen; can use it to control heart rate.	daily	Box breathing technique counsellor suggested. Also Functional Medicine practitioner sent me a link.
Cold water on neck	Feel more alert, like my brain is working properly.	daily	Maybe try cold water immersion?
Acupuncture	Full-body healing as well as symptom-specific.	every 3 weeks	Have changed frequency as health improves (began with weekly sessions).

My Full-Body Healing Strategies (cont.)

Strategy	How it works for me	Frequency	Resources/notes

Symptom Causes

You will notice that I have not mentioned anything about specific *causes* of our symptoms. This is intentional. Some of us are about a year into living with this, and we still don't have any specific explanations for many of our strange symptoms — all we really know is that they started after vaccination. Some of us have given up trying to get to the bottom of what's causing them, and some of us are still battling away. Until someone in the medical profession starts doing actual research, we are, quite simply, not going to get any real answers, as hard as that is for us to accept, and as unfair as it may be.

I've always been the kind of person who has wanted to get to the bottom of any health issues — I'm not a fan of being patched up and sent away. I want to understand *why* something happened and know how to prevent it happening again. To work out what I can do to help myself. This approach of needing to understand *why* does not work in the situation I now find myself in, and, when I've become a little too focused on the cause of one symptom or another, it has actually interfered with my ongoing recovery. A lot of us feel the same.

So for this particular, very complicated health condition, I truly believe that our best approach to symptom management is to accept that, right now, the answers we need simply aren't there, but this doesn't mean that we can't tackle our symptoms one at a time, while also doing what we can to support full-body healing.

This entire book is not focused on looking at *causes*, but is instead focused on looking at contributing factors. Factors that may or may not have contributed to the situation we now find ourselves in; factors that can make us feel absolutely terrible for days, weeks, or months on end; factors that contribute to our ongoing healing and recovery; and factors that we may at some point make a decision we want to continue with. If we look at contributing factors in this way, then this entire experience feels less overwhelming, and much, much more manageable. It feels like something that we have at least some level of control over.

In taking control of our own symptom management, we are less emotionally invested in the doctors or specialists that we previously believed would be able to help us. So when they tell us they don't know, or there's nothing they can do, then we don't get upset. Instead we simply shrug, confident that we will figure this out ourselves.

Wheel of Healing Update

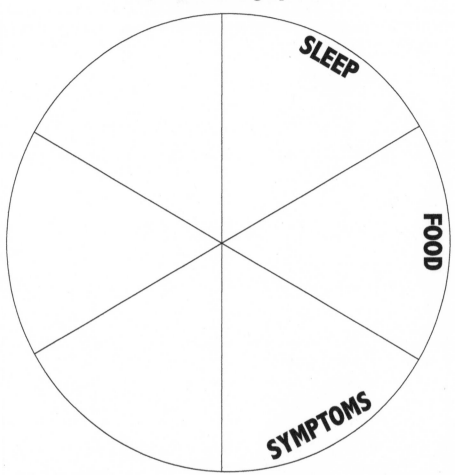

Before you add your actions for dealing with your symptoms, first take a moment to update your Sleep actions. Ask yourself whether your sleep has improved. Does it need a bit more effort? Or have you managed to achieve a sleep pattern that is maximising your recovery? And your diet ... what's your focus right now? What do you need to eat more or less of? Is there a nutrition programme that you want to try at this stage of your recovery?

Then, in the Symptoms section, make some notes on what specific symptoms you want to focus on first, as well as a couple of full-body healing techniques you'd like to try. Don't try to tackle too much at once.

My Symptom Resources (books/websites/articles)

Other Notes/Thoughts on Symptoms

Before you start this chapter ...

This entire chapter is dedicated to dealing with what, for some, may be a highly challenging topic. There are exercises here that may trigger difficult memories. If you are working with a counsellor, then I'd recommend asking them to work through this chapter with you. If you're dealing with this alone, then take this chapter very slowly, give yourself lots of time in between topics, and just skip anything that you feel unable to handle. Come back to it when you feel ready.

CHAPTER 4: STRESS

SUMMARY

We have dealt with stress/pressure in the past and overcome it.
Stress has become a dismissive explanation for many health issues.
Our bodies have a real and powerful physical response to stress.
We can learn techniques to control that physical response.
Those techniques can help us live life without fear.

One very important contributing factor that I did not mention in the previous chapter is "stress." Is it a symptom? Is it what lies behind our symptoms? Or is it a result of our symptoms? Is it historically relevant? Is it relevant at all? How does it feature in our future now that we have all these health challenges to deal with? "Stress" is such a huge topic in itself, and I believe it is relevant to people like us on a number of very complicated and interconnected levels.

"Stress" is possibly the one area over which we potentially have so much more power than we realise. But for many of us it feels like the most difficult to understand and the most difficult to manage. So in this chapter, I want to really simplify this topic. I want to break it all down, with language that all of us can understand, without the need for a degree in psychotherapy.

Just talking about "stress" can ironically make us feel even more stressed, and I hope that, by reexamining how we look at "stress," it will become much easier to manage. I hope that the whole concept of stress becomes less BIG and overwhelming, and instead that dealing with it becomes something as simple as eating more leafy greens. To do that, let's look at how we define "stress" and the role it played in our lives before the vaccine.

Defining "Stress"

Most accepted definitions generally refer to stress being a form of pressure or tension. Some definitions include an element of feeling unable to cope with that pressure. Some definitions refer to the pressure itself being the stress, and some definitions refer to our *response* to the pressure as being the stress — the *feeling* of being stressed.

Throughout our lives, we will already have experienced times when we have felt under pressure. One little exercise that may be helpful is to take some time to think back on those times and to try to remember how we dealt with them.

Pressures In the Past

I was under pressure when ...	I dealt with it by ...

Reminding ourselves of times in our past when we have been under pressure (or have been stressed), is a really good exercise in reminding ourselves of how we coped. And the fact that we *did* cope.

We found some ways of coping with that pressure, and managed to live through those experiences. We have already developed some skills to draw upon to help get through this current challenge. We have done this before and we can do it now.

Use of the Word "Stress" in Medical Conversations

The word "stress" can be a trigger word for many people who have a history of complicated health problems, myself included. If this is not your first time dealing with inexplicable symptoms, then you will probably have had the word stress thrown at you more than a few times in the past. If this is your first complex medical situation, get used to hearing it.

I feel like stress has become the go-to word for lazy medical professionals to use in order to dismiss symptoms that they do not understand and have no interest or ability in pursuing further. And those lazy professionals seem to have an incredible talent for delivering a "stress diagnosis" in a way that makes you somehow feel inadequate for no longer being able to manage your life in the way you used to. It is often delivered with no explanation of what *pressure* does to your body from a physiological point of view, and no treatment plan other than to "take some time off work." You take the time off, and do feel better for it, but the relief is short-lived and, as soon as you're back at work, your symptoms flare up again.

Life presents us with people and circumstances that have the potential to create pressure in our lives. It can come from our parents, our kids, our friends, our work, having some building work done on the house, a political situation, being stuck in traffic, being late, giving a presentation, or meeting a deadline. It is virtually impossible to remove or control any potential source of pressure. Dealing with a complex medical condition, that nobody seems to understand, that changes day by day, and that has completely disrupted your entire life, is a *very* high-pressure situation. And every single one of us has felt like we absolutely cannot cope.

It is *completely normal* to be overwhelmed in this situation. Our feelings are a totally normal response to a possibly life-threatening and definitely life-changing event.

But this particular event in our lives is not going to magically go away on its own anytime soon, so we must take responsibility for how we handle the pressure we feel under to deal with it. We have to find ways of dealing with that pressure. Not to *fight* the pressure, but to feel it, acknowledge it, embrace it, and move *with* it.

For me, learning about how pressure physically affects my body, at a time when I am entirely focused on and committed to recovery, has been a huge motivation to never, ever let "stress" affect me again.

How Our Bodies Respond to Pressure

Take a moment to think about what physically happens in your body when you feel under pressure. How do you feel if you have to speak in public? What about when you see a family member you find toxic? When you have to make a very difficult phone call to someone?

What actually happens in your body at those times? Go through every part of your body, from head to toe, and identify what each part feels like. How does it change from when you are not feeling under pressure? I have three very clear things that happen to me: my heart starts beating really fast; I start sweating under my armpits, but the sweat smells different to normal sweat; and I find myself needing a massive poo. What happens to you?

My Body's Physical Response to Pressure

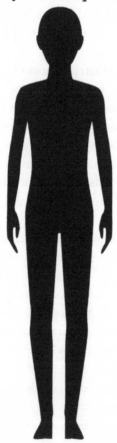

WHY Our Bodies Respond to Pressure

Our bodies respond the way they do when under pressure because they think they're under attack. Every physical response is designed to enable us to stand up to a threat, run away from one, or stop dead in our tracks so we are not perceived to be a threat ourselves. My heart starts pumping faster in order to get oxygen to my limbs to make them work faster; my sweat smells different because it's been triggered by adrenaline, which will give me more energy; and I suddenly need that massive poo because my body wants to be as light as possible to maximise efficiency. Whatever different ways our different bodies respond to pressure, they have one thing in common: they are literally preparing to fight, take flight, or freeze. That "stress" response — it's trying to save our lives.

But our bodies are not designed to respond to pressure in this way very often. Responding to pressure creates pressure of its own. My heart is not supposed to be beating that fast, my liver is not supposed to constantly detox from adrenaline, and my gut needs hours to process food in a way that will nourish me. We are not supposed to go into "life-saving" mode on a regular basis.

Historical Trauma

Some of us have a very, very long history of going into that life-saving mode. Some of us have been exposed to so much pressure in our lifetimes that we may have developed a habit of always being just a little bit alert. Or we may have experienced pressure resulting from a deeply distressing event or events considered to be "trauma." Perhaps we have been unlucky enough to suffer from more than one trauma in our lifetime. And if we grew up in an environment where we experienced pressure or trauma as a normal part of life, then our bodies have developed with life-saving mode as our default. We may have lived life with our bodies always ready to deal with a life-threatening situation, even when one did not exist. We don't know how to *not* be on alert.

Our body's ability to protect us by being ready to fight, take flight, or freeze may have served us well on the odd occasion in the past, but it is greatly affecting our ability to heal right now. We must come out of life-saving mode in order to give our bodies the best possible chance to recover.

This realisation was a *huge* wake-up call for me. And enough of a motivation to learn exactly what my triggers are, and how to control my body's response.

Pressure Situations

You can use the chart below to note the kinds of situations that seem to trigger your body's physical response to pressure. You might already know of some things to put here, or you might find that you add to this chart over time. Some might be avoidable. Some may not.

When I first did this, I identified a number of situations that always seemed to get my heart racing: whenever I had a medical appointment, whenever I had to call any customer service representatives, and whenever I had to speak to a certain family member. The first two situations were unavoidable, but I avoided the third while I was learning how to deal with my body's response to pressure.

For now, complete the first two columns of the chart. We'll address the right hand column later.

My Pressure Situations

Situation	Avoidable? Y/N	Body's response managed!

Controlling Your Body's Response

You could embark on some really intensive therapy to deal with your body's response to pressure, which may well be incredibly helpful as you deal with this entire vaccine-related experience. Therapy can be life-changing. However, you may not have the funds or the inclination to explore traumatic events in your past that may be contributing to an especially active response to pressure. There is enough going on for you at the moment, and you may not want to delve deeply into unpleasant memories. But what you *can* do, entirely on your own, is learn to control your body's physical response. I have three things that are incredibly effective for me, that took me just a few days to learn:

- **Breathing:** Very deep breathing — in to the count of ten, and out to the same count. As soon as I feel my heart speed up, I stop whatever I am doing or thinking, and immediately breathe this way, focusing on slowing my heart rate. It works every time.

- **Nurturing excitement:** If I notice strange-smelling sweat under my arms and I'm giving a speech that day, then I know that, whether I'm aware of it or not, I'm feeling nervous. Knowing this, I say out loud, in between deep breaths, "This is exciting!" I once read about anxiety and excitement provoking the same physical responses, but if you *tell* your body that something positive is about to happen, then it changes the impact of that experience on your body from one of pressure to one of joy.

- **Reassurance:** This is my favourite one because its effectiveness surprised me. Depending on the situation that's started my heart racing (it's especially effective if I'm feeling anxious about having to interact with someone I don't want to interact with, like a medical professional), I will say out loud in between deep breaths, "I am safe. I am safe. I am safe."

There are lots of other techniques you can use to try to control your body's physical response to pressure. Some are techniques that you can spend months, if not years, perfecting, but to be quite honest I think we need a few little tools, right now, that we can *instantly* draw upon in any situation, that we know will work within minutes. Use the next page to make notes on some techniques you want to try out, see how they work for you, and then go back to the chart on the opposite page and note when you've learned how to manage your body's response to a particular situation. Congratulate yourself!

Techniques to Control My Body's Response to Pressure

Technique	How To Do It	Results/Notes

Fear

As I learned about the impact of stress on my body, and experimented with different ways to control my body's response to it, I started looking at stress in quite a different way. I started to look at it in terms of *fear*. There were two reasons I started looking at stress in this way.

First, I thought about how the fight, flight, or freeze responses occur when animals feel *afraid*. They become aware of a threat and instinctively choose an appropriate response depending on the level of fear they might be feeling. Their subsequent actions (or inaction) are a direct response to being afraid. This got me thinking about what I might be afraid of in those moments when my heart starts racing. Why on earth would I be experiencing *fear* when making a phone call to my doctor's surgery? (Note: for what it's worth, I don't think it's necessary to be able to answer *why* we're experiencing fear in order to move forward with healing. Just the act of perceiving stress in terms of fear is enough. But in my case, I assumed that the fear of calling my doctor's surgery was rooted in historical medical gaslighting from a different medical practice.)

Second, the action of repeating, "I am safe. I am safe. I am safe." to myself in those times of "stress" *astounded* me with how effective it was. Was that all it took? I just needed somebody to tell me that I was safe? The more I thought about it, the more I realised it made sense. We are dealing with a complicated health condition that no one seems able to explain, alleviate, or solve. Of course we don't feel safe right now. And if you compound that with growing up in an "unsafe" environment, being in an "unsafe" relationship, or dealing with an "unsafe" medical situation in the past, then for some of us, the world in general probably hasn't felt like a safe place for a very long time. And that means a lot of healing is required.

So in order to protect our body so that it can focus on healing and recovery, we have to send it the message that it is safe. That we are safe. To reassure ourselves on a deep level that, right now, in this very moment, we are safe. It actually doesn't matter whether it's true or not. It matters that we *believe* it's true. Try saying it *out loud* until you feel your body relax, your thoughts become calm, and a smile emerge. Say it as often as you need to until you feel the fear leave your body. Say it every time you feel yourself under stress or pressure. Tell yourself that the world is a safe place for you. I will tell you — you are safe.

What Are We Afraid Of?

For some of us, all we may need to do when we feel the physical impact of stress in our bodies is to tell ourselves that we are safe. Just those three simple words may be enough. But some of us might want to delve a little deeper into those feelings of fear.

Of the emails and private messages I receive from other people who are also dealing with adverse reactions, I'd say that more than ninety percent contain the words "I am afraid of ..." or "I am worried about ..." at some point. Sometimes they don't even say *what* they are worried about or afraid of, but they very clearly express that they are feeling scared. Some people regularly contact me and tell me exactly the same thing each time — their fear is ongoing to the point where they are afraid of their feelings of fear.

I think it can be really helpful for us to stop fighting those feelings and thoughts, and to stay with them, identify them, and express them on paper. To try not to *fear* fear, if you like. Give it a voice. And keep it simple.

I'm not afraid anymore but, when I was, these are some of the things I was afraid of:
- Not being able to write again.
- Not being able to walk again.
- Not being able to work again.
- Losing my business.
- Losing my relationship.
- Losing my home.
- Losing *me*.

That last one makes me feel emotional just typing it, so clearly that was the one I was most afraid of, and perhaps I still carry a bit of fear in that one. It's also the fear that I see regularly expressed among many of us — we are afraid that at our core, we are not the same anymore, and that we never will be again.

Use the next page to try to identify what exactly you feel afraid of right now. Try to get as many fears out as you can. It doesn't have to just be about your health or even personal to your situation. I know that, in addition to the above, for a long time I had a general feeling of *fear* relating to humanity, the world, and my place in it as a vaccine-injured person. Some of us will be afraid of the bigger picture.

What Am I Afraid Of?

Dealing with Fear

If all you need to do is learn some techniques to control your body's response to stress/pressure/fear, then that's fine. If it's not too difficult emotionally, then the space on the previous page for you to make notes on what you're afraid of might be helpful. And you can leave it at that. You've taken two huge steps that will greatly aid your recovery. You can skip to the end of this chapter.

Or, you can take control of your response to the fear not just from a physical perspective but from psychological and emotional perspectives, too. You can have a really strong word with yourself. Maybe even dare, as well, to find some humour while having that strong word? For example, at one point in the early months I remember feeling terrified and utterly consumed with fear about what the future held for me. I was standing in the kitchen crying and crying at my boyfriend as I blurted out one thing after another that I was scared about. At one point I wailed, "What will we do if I end up in a wheelchair?!" and he responded very calmly but with a huge grin, "Then I'll get one too and we'll have races." That statement immediately stopped my catastrophic thinking, and the image of the two of us racing around our town made me giggle. From that moment, I started making a real effort to teach myself to do that.

On the next page you can take some of your fears and make notes on some completely different ways of looking at them. Try to think outside the box. What is the silliest response you might have to yourself? Try to open your mind enough to envision *advantages* if that fear actually comes true! By doing this, you might find that you can persuade some of those fears to occupy just a little less space in your life. This is a way for you to focus more on healing.

I like the approach above because there is so much room for humour but, now that I've got to a point where fear no longer dominates my recovery, I use much simpler and more well-known techniques, techniques that return my focus to living in the moment, to halt in their tracks any "what if" thoughts. For me this literally involves saying to myself, "What am I doing right now?" and I have learned to apply it to all sorts of thoughts that my mind might run away with. My thought process goes like this: I realise that I'm thinking rather a lot and feeling a little anxious about a medical appointment with a new specialist next week. I tell myself to STOP. I ask myself, "What am I *actually* doing right now?" And as I'm chopping some vegetables for some soup, I think only about that.

My fear	My current train of thought regarding it	Other ways of looking at it (include fun, crazy, positive ways too)

Your Future Relationship with Fear

You're probably already realising that many elements of your recovery will have an impact on your future far beyond the adverse reaction. It is my hope that this book will help you to learn new ways of managing a deeply traumatic event and to acquire skills that will be useful for the rest of your life. The tools we learn *now* to deal with stress or pressure or fear — whatever you want to call it — may be invaluable for years to come.

We may have grown up with fear all around us. Some of us come from families where keeping ourselves safe — physically and/or emotionally — was our priority because the adults around us did not make it theirs. We became highly sensitive to our environments, which perhaps made us highly sensitive to people in general, not just those in our families. This level of empathy is a truly wonderful quality, and I have seen it in a lot of the new friends I've made throughout the world during this experience, but it also makes us very sensitive to the collective pain that everyone has been dealing with since early 2020. We have been living through *extremely* difficult times, on a global scale. And now some of the most sensitive among us are dealing with vaccine injuries.

Covid aside, we have spent *years* living in a world where stress or pressure is part of our everyday lives in ways that our bodies were never designed for. We are not taught what stress actually means, we are not taught how our bodies respond to it and why, and we are not taught about the very real physical impact of stress *on* our bodies over an extended period of time.

We have to make dealing with stress/pressure/fear an important part of our ongoing recovery plan, and learn about tools that will become habits.

We need to make a very conscious decision not to live in fear.

Wheel of Healing Update

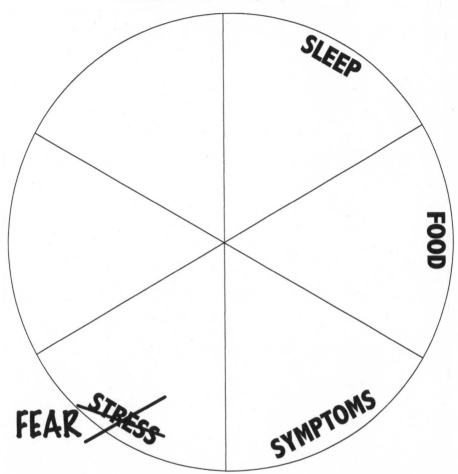

Before you add your actions for dealing with your fears, first take a moment to update your Sleep, Food, and Symptoms actions. How are you sleeping now? Is there anything you can do to improve it? And your diet ... do you need to cut out anything? Eat more of something else? Is there anything that might make your food preparation or management a little easier? Which symptom is bothering you the most at the moment? Are you thinking about adding a specific full-body healing technique to your current efforts?

Then, in the Fear section, maybe note one of the techniques you want to try to use to control your body's response, and make practising that your focus for a while.

My Stress/Fear Resources (books/websites/articles)

Other Notes/Thoughts on Stress/Fear

Before you start this chapter ...

You may already have felt let down by professionals you *assumed* would be available to guide you through this challenging and distressing health experience. It's a big shock at first and I feel for you. Use the space above to keep track of those people so you can move on and away from them. The people you list above are not going to help you in your efforts to recover. This chapter is designed to help you identify the professionals who will.

CHAPTER 5: CONSULTANTS

SUMMARY

We go to consultants for information — it is up to us what we do with it.
State-affiliated health consultants are limited in what they can offer us.
Consultants can be organ/system-specific or focused on full-body healing.
Be prepared to be told it's all in our heads (numerous times).
Our healing is not diagnosis-dependent.

In this chapter, I use the word "consultants" to refer to anyone who is trained in a specific area of healthcare, and may be able to offer us some level of support in our recovery. But before looking at these consultants, I think it is important to remind ourselves of what exactly "consult" means, and why this definition is vital to us when dealing with such a complicated situation.

The general definition of "consult" is to seek information or advice from someone with specialist knowledge. It does not mean to get *definitive* answers, treatment, or instructions. It does not mean that you have to follow or even believe everything that consultant says. It just means that you are communicating with them for the purpose of gathering information. *You* make the decisions.

There are no consultants who treat adverse reactions to the Covid vaccine. There is no one person we can go to who will have any answers, let alone all of them. There are very few people actively working in the field, and those that are are not being very public about it. It is simply too early — the vaccine has not been around for long enough for there to be any consultants with specialist knowledge in this area. And it is too controversial — to consult on vaccine adverse reactions means to admit that they exist.

We are in a situation where we are dealing with a very new medical condition, so no long-term data is available, and it is affecting our bodies in a variety of different ways. No one is (yet) researching how to treat us, so we have to find a way to work with what we have.

The consultants we can access fall under two healthcare categories: I'll call them (1) state-affiliated and (2) independent. This probably sounds obvious but, just to be clear ... wherever you are in the world, for the purposes of this book, if I'm referring to state-affiliated consultants then I'm talking about the consultants that are available through your country's approved or provided health services. In the UK, the state-affiliated consultants are working within the free National Health Service (NHS) and also within the fee-paying private sector while following NHS guidelines.

Again, this may seem obvious but, for clarity, when I say "independent" consultants, I am referring to specialists who work outside your country's approved or provided health services. These consultants may have membership in or affiliation with professional bodies relevant to their field of expertise. There may be a little overlap; for example, some consultants might be NHS-trained and work in an NHS hospital, but perhaps run their own private clinic in which you can get an appointment entirely independent of the NHS. The key difference is that the independent consultants are able to provide information and advice *outside* of what the NHS guidelines permit.

The most important thing to understand is that any state-affiliated consultants will have to follow national guidelines on the information, advice, and treatment that they are *allowed* to give you. Their ability to consult is limited to whatever is in those guidelines. So when they seem unable to help, it is not because help is not available, and it is not necessarily because they don't *want* to help you; it is because they do not have any way to help you *through the system they are affiliated with*. If you are being diagnosed with mental health issues, then that is because your symptoms match mental health conditions *according to their system*. If you're a woman over forty, then those very same symptoms will check a lot of boxes for menopause, according to their system — so that's what you'll be "treated" for.

The following pages give descriptions of some of the professionals that you may choose to consult with, and ways they might be able to support you.

Consultant	Area of expertise	Possibly helpful for (in the context of vaccine recovery)
Acupuncturist	Traditional Chinese medicine that involves inserting fine needles into certain parts of the body for the purpose of regulating the flow of the patient's "life energy."	General pain relief, improving blood flow, symptom-specific relief, full-body healing.
Biofeedback Therapist	The use of information from the body (such as breathing patterns, temperature, heart rate, muscle tension) to teach patients how to control their body. (Neurofeedback uses only brain activity.)	Anxiety, pain, blood pressure, tinnitus, circulation problems.
Cardiologist	All areas of heart health including blood vessels in the heart.	Diagnosis, treatment, and management of conditions affecting the heart. Testing for physical heart defects, blood flow problems, or how well the heart is functioning.
Chiropractor	Problems relating to bones, muscles, and joints, and how to relieve them through manipulation of the spine.	Pain relief, injuries, sleep problems.
Counsellor	Identifying emotional issues that are causing problems in day-to-day living.	Finding solutions to problem-causing issues, and ways to cope with their impact.
Craniosacral Therapist	Light touching, mainly around the head and neck, to release tension in the body and promote overall healing.	Relief of stress and tension. Pain relief especially in the head, neck, ear, and back areas.

Consultant	Area of expertise	Possibly helpful for (in the context of vaccine recovery)
Functional Medicine Practitioner	Identifying root causes of complex illness with respect to environmental, historical, physical, and emotional contributing factors, and developing personalised treatment plans.	Developing nutrition, supplement, and lifestyle changes to maximise recovery; gut health testing.
Gastroenterologist	Gastrointestinal (GI) issues, the digestive system: stomach, intestine, liver, gallbladder, pancreas.	Test, diagnose, treat, and manage GI problems or diseases. Check how well food is moving through the body. Test gut microbes. Look for causes of diarrhea.
GP/PCP (General Practitioner/ Primary Care Practitioner)	Common medical conditions.	Providing access to specialists, arranging standard blood tests, following up after emergency medical care, administrative support (e.g., providing vaccine exemptions, sick notes for employers, documents for insurance).
Haematologist	Blood.	Diagnosis, treatment, and management of blood disorders. Blood and bone marrow testing. Examination of organs involved in blood production.
Homeopath	250-year-old practice of treating an ailment with a small amount of what caused the ailment in the first place. Uses natural substances to promote the body's natural healing ability.	Treatment of minor ailments such as coughs and colds, and more complicated long-term conditions that affect the whole body either physically or emotionally.
Immunologist	The immune system. Allergies.	Diagnosis and treatment of conditions brought about by a very active immune system (e.g., asthma, food sensitivities, sinus problems, skin problems). Can help identify triggers.

Consultant	Area of expertise	Possibly helpful for (in the context of vaccine recovery)
Lymphatic Massage Therapist	Gentle massage to stimulate the removal of toxins via the lymphatic drainage system.	Dissolution of swelling in lymph nodes, general detoxification, sinus blockage relief, inflammation reduction.
Naturopath	Natural remedies to encourage the body to heal itself.	Diagnosing underlying causes of health problems (physical or emotional), recommending natural healing methods to stimulate the body's natural healing ability.
Neurologist	The brain and spinal cord, and parts of the body (such as nerves and muscles) involved in the functioning of the two.	Diagnosis, treatment, and management of strokes, multiple sclerosis, brain infections, seizures, degenerative brain disease, and other conditions causing headaches, migraines, nerve pain, memory loss, tremors.
Neuropsychologist	How physical changes in or diseases of the brain are related to changes in cognitive functions and behaviour.	Diagnosis, treatment, and management of brain injuries, brain diseases such as Parkinson's and Alzheimer's, or mental health conditions such as depression and anxiety. Development of coping mechanisms.
Nutritionist	The impact of food on health.	Development of diet and meal plans to promote healthy eating or for the purpose of recovery from specific conditions.
Ophthalmologist	Eye disorders and visual problems.	Diagnosis, treatment, and management of conditions such as diabetes, high blood pressure, high cholesterol, cancer, multiple sclerosis, thyroid disease, lupus, rheumatoid arthritis, sexually transmitted diseases, Lyme disease, and brain tumours.

Consultant	Area of expertise	Possibly helpful for (in the context of vaccine recovery)
Osteopath	Moving, stretching, and massaging of bones and muscles for the purpose of returning the body to its natural state and promoting overall body healing.	Relief of problems with or pain in the joints, back, and neck.
Otolaryngologist (ENT specialist)	Head and neck problems, including ear, nose, and throat.	Diagnosis, treatment, and management of hearing loss, tinnitus, balance problems, nerve pain, and head and neck disorders such as Bell's palsy (a type of paralysis affecting one side of the face).
Phlebotomist	Taking blood.	Improvement of cognitive function and energy levels.
Psychiatrist	Mental illnesses.	Diagnosis, treatment, and management of mental health conditions. (I only include this here because vaccine-injured people may receive referrals to psychiatrists and NOT because I think they are relevant or useful to us — this is not a mental illness.)
Psychologist	Behaviour, thoughts, and emotions.	Developing strategies for dealing with the mental health impact of a physical health condition.
Psychotherapist	Understanding how past experiences and patterns of behaviour may be affecting historical, current, and future wellbeing.	Depression, anxiety, dealing with subconscious challenges, increased understanding of the psychological impact of dealing with a physical health challenge.

Consultant	Area of expertise	Possibly helpful for (in the context of vaccine recovery)
Pulmonologist	The respiratory system (from the nose to the blood vessels in the lungs).	Diagnosis, treatment, and management of bronchitis, chronic obstructive pulmonary disease (COPD), and sleep disorders affecting breathing. Testing for possible causes of shortness of breath.
Reflexology	Applying pressure to specific parts of the foot in order to stimulate healing in a related part of the body.	Stimulating healing in a specific part of the body or system-wide, improving circulation, pain relief.
Reiki Practitioner	Japanese practice of non-contact energy healing.	Insomnia, stress, pain, anxiety, depression, promoting the body's ability to heal itself.
Respirologist	The treatment of lung disease.	Diagnosis, treatment, and management of lung diseases. Testing for breathing problems.
Rheumatologist	Joints, bones, muscles, and their connected tissues.	Diagnosis, treatment, and management of inflammatory/degenerative joint diseases, autoimmune disease, bone problems.
Vascular Surgeon	Veins, arteries, and anything to do with blood vessels, excluding the heart and brain.	Diagnosis, treatment, and management of circulation problems and blood vessel disease.

"Unhelpful" General Practitioners

We would do well to remind ourselves that general health practitioners are not specialists. They are extremely limited in what they might be able to do in order to help us, for a number of reasons:

- We are experiencing a very complicated health condition that affects our bodies in a range of quite different and seemingly unrelated ways. General practitioners are not trained to deal with complex conditions such as ours, and they may not have had much experience of them in the past. Our conditions may baffle them as much as us and they may genuinely have no idea what to do.

- Covid itself is a new disease. Our symptoms may be very similar to those of people dealing with Long Covid, but general practitioners don't know what to do with Long Covid sufferers either; the condition that most closely resembles our own is not yet understood either.

- The Covid vaccines are also new and there is still very limited research into side effects and adverse reactions. Therefore, there is not yet enough data on potential *treatments* for adverse reactions. Most of our general practitioners will never have (knowingly) come across adverse reactions to vaccinations or perhaps even to medications in general, so, again, they may genuinely have absolutely no idea what to do.

For the sake of our mental health, and to make interactions with our general practitioners much less stressful, we need to remind ourselves that they do not have any answers, because the answers simply don't exist yet.

None of the above are excuses for being dismissed, or for being treated unkindly by your general practitioner. There are no excuses for someone working in healthcare to be anything but caring, but we know that some can be quite unhelpful. If your general practitioner is not being *kind* when you ask them for help, then request another one, ask for a second opinion, make a formal complaint, or stop asking them for help. We have to stop expecting kindness from someone who clearly is unwilling to give it. With that attitude, these practitioners are never going to be part of our recovery. We have to accept that, however hard it is. Write their name on the page preceding this chapter, and move on to someone who will at least be kind.

What General Practitioners CAN Help With

For some of us, general practitioners are the gatekeepers to our country's entire medical system, and it is important that we understand their role within it, specifically when our health conditions become complicated. Here is what a general practitioner will be able to help us with:

- **Tests:** Whether it is blood, wee, or poo, a GP can get it tested. *But*, they must have a reason to get it tested, so, if you don't tick one of the boxes for a specific test, they can't request it, or, if they do, that request can be declined if the reason isn't good enough. The decision to test will not necessarily be theirs. And the more specific a test is, the less likely they'll even have access to someone who can carry out that test. It is not as simple as just requesting a test from your GP and getting it done. If you can't get your GP to arrange for the tests you want, then you will have to go private.
- **Referrals:** If you need access to a specialist, it's likely that you will need your GP's cooperation, especially if you're hoping to see a state-funded specialist (but, in many cases, also if you're seeing someone privately). A GP will be able to write directly to the specialist to request that they see you but, again, the specialist may refuse despite your GP's support. You need to tick certain boxes not just to get the referral, but to get the referral *accepted*.
- **Admin:** Your GP can provide sick notes for your employer, and reports for any private insurance plans you may have. In the UK they are also expected to tick the boxes required for vaccine exemption applications but they do *not* make the decision of whether those applications are successful or not.
- **Prescriptions:** Your GP can write you a prescription for medication and supplements from an approved list. Some medications you read about may not be approved in your country.

We need to find a way to "use" our GPs and the limitations imposed on them by the medical system within which they work so that we can move forward with our recovery. Tests, Referrals, Admin, and Prescriptions (TRAP) are all important parts of that and we need to learn to keep our GP interactions focused on those things, instead of falling into the *trap* of thinking they have all the answers and are capable of fixing us. They are not. We need to carefully prepare for GP appointments in order to stay focused on making the limited time spent with them worthwhile.

Managing Your GP/PCP Appointment

It helps both us and them if we try to work not just within their medical system, but also within their time constraints.

- Find out how long your appointment is for and ask for a double appointment if you don't feel that it's long enough.
- Keep your eye on the time and aim to finish within that time, unless they indicate that you can go on for longer.
- Take a copy of the diagram of all your symptoms. Highlight the one/ones you specifically want to discuss and stick to that.
- Keep your conversation focused on the four things they can do — Tests, Referrals, Admin, Prescriptions — and remind yourself not to fall into the *trap* of thinking they can do anything else.
- If you run out of time, book another appointment.

We need to find a general practitioner that we can get along with. They cannot change anything about the system in which they work. But we can change how we work with them. We need to be OK with them not having all the answers. We need to be patient. And we need to become a patient that they enjoy speaking to and end up really wanting to help.

General Practitioner/Primary Care Practitioner Appointment Record Example	
Doctor	**Reminder!** Don't fall into the TRAP of thinking they have all the answers
Doctor Name	**Reason for appointment:** Show symptom chart/focus on one specific symptom
Clinic	**Tests:** What tests do they have access to that might be relevant? Are there
Clinic Name	any other tests that I could have done privately, and if so, how do I go about
Date	arranging for them to be done?
14 Feb 2022	**Referrals:** What specialists would they recommend I see? How long might the waiting list be? What private consultants could I be looking at?
Time	**Admin:** Request sick note. Is there any financial or practical support available that I should be aware of? How do I apply for a vaccine exemption?
12:15pm	**Prescriptions:** What medication or supplements can they prescribe that might
Duration	help? Is there anything available that they cannot prescribe to deal with this symptom? Where would I find more information about that?
7 minutes	
Kind/Helpful	**Next step:** Do I feel comfortable consulting with them again? How would they like me to share with them any new research I may come across? Based on how this
yes/no	appointment went, what do I want to do next? Remember it is MY choice.

General Practitioner/Primary Care Practitioner Appointment Record	
Doctor	**Reminder!** Don't fall into the TRAP of thinking they have all the answers
	Reason for appointment:
Clinic	
	Tests:
Date	
	Referrals:
Time	
	Admin:
Duration	
	Prescriptions:
Kind/Helpful	
	Next step:

General Practitioner/Primary Care Practitioner Appointment Record	
Doctor	**Reminder!** Don't fall into the TRAP of thinking they have all the answers
	Reason for appointment:
Clinic	
	Tests:
Date	
	Referrals:
Time	
	Admin:
Duration	
	Prescriptions:
Kind/Helpful	
	Next step:

The Other Consultants

You will have noticed that the *non*-general practitioner consultants listed on the earlier pages of this chapter tend to fall into two categories: organ- or system-specific health, and general full-body health. There are some basic differences between the two that can be helpful for us to know.

We tend to be able to access the organ/system-specific consultants via our national health systems, whereas most of the full-body consultants are independent. There is a little overlap among both, and the organ/system-specific consultants often have private practices, but, for the most part, to access the organ/system-specific consultants we need cooperation from a GP/PCP who is working within our country's national health system.

Organ/system-specific consultants will only focus on a specific part of the body. As a rule, they will not look at what is going on in any other organs or systems within the body, whereas full-body health consultants will look at what is going on throughout the whole body.

Organ/system-specific consultants will generally have a procedure to follow that includes conducting certain tests to either diagnose or rule out specific conditions or diseases that are directly related to a single organ or system. Symptom A results in Test B, which will either diagnose or rule out Condition C. If Condition C is diagnosed, then Treatment D is recommended. If Test B rules out Condition C and there are no more tests on their list then they have done their job and there is nothing more they can do. Full-body health consultants are not so focused on one specific symptom or one specific part of the body — they are more focused on the whole person and what they can to do heal the whole body.

Organ/system-specific consultants tend to be working within a strict time allocation, which would be longer than a GP/PCP appointment but is still relatively short (perhaps 30 minutes), whereas full-body health consultants tend to spend around an hour with you per session, and we often see them for multiple sessions over several months.

These big differences mean that, like the general practitioners, many of the organ/system-specific consultants are simply not able to deal with complex health conditions that affect multiple organs and systems. The healthcare system within which they work does not teach them to connect the dots and we need to accept this. According to *their* system, there is nothing wrong with us. Some consultants will directly (and sometimes what feels like harshly) tell us that there is nothing wrong with us, and some will be more accurate and say that they cannot *find* anything wrong with us. This is a very big difference, and one that we need to remind ourselves of when we are feeling despondent after an appointment with a specialist that we tried so hard and waited so long to get in front of.

Having someone say, "There's nothing wrong with you" does not bring about the relief that others might expect. It doesn't change anything about how truly awful we feel. If anything, it can sometimes make us feel worse because we feel dismissed, unheard, and lost, especially if the lack of a diagnosis is delivered without compassion or a plan for a next step. Time and time again, it feels like we are getting nowhere in our search for answers to the question, "What is wrong with me?" So we need to change the question we are asking.

"What Is Wrong With Me?" Versus "How Do I Heal?"

This is where the full-body health consultants can be invaluable. They tend not to see us as having something "wrong" with us that needs fixing. They tend to see us as rounded people with rich, complex lives that have been dramatically affected by trauma. That trauma may be physical, psychological, or both; it may be historical or current; and it may be affecting our entire body in all sorts of complicated ways that are hindering our ability to function as we used to. Right now, the trauma that is requiring our urgent attention is an adverse reaction to a vaccine, but the full-body health consultants are interested in helping us heal not just from that, but from all sorts of other trauma that may or may not be affecting us now or have affected us in the past.

In order to find out about our whole bodies and whole lives, these kinds of consultants need and want to spend *time* with us. They want to listen to our symptoms and how they make us feel. They want to know how we are coping. They want to understand how a vaccine injury affects different parts of our lives. And even on its own, their act of listening, hearing, accepting, and validating can bring about incredible healing. Spending time talking with a healthcare consultant who makes us feel like they actually *care* about our recovery and actively want to be a part of it makes us feel completely different from spending time with one who isn't really interested but will run some tests — that's not how we *heal*.

Organ/System-Specific Consultant Appointment Record	
Consultant	**Organ/System:**
	DURING THE APPOINTMENT **Organ/System-specific symptoms:**
Practice	**Possible explanations:**
	Available tests:
Date	
	Other investigations:
Time	**When results will be available:**
	UPON RECEIPT OF RESULTS **Results indicate:**
Duration	**Diagnosis:**
	Treatment plan:
Kind/Helpful	**Other next steps:**

Full-Body Consultant Appointment Record	
Consultant	NOTE: Your diagram of all your symptoms will be very helpful for these appointments. Don't forget to show them it!
	Topics explored that might explain symptoms:
Expertise	
	Recommended testing:
Practice Name	
	Nutritional recommendations:
Date	
	Other healing therapies recommended:
Time	
	Treatments used during session:
Duration	
	Impact of treatments in the hours/days/weeks that followed:
Kind/Helpful	
	Next appointment:

Overview of Consultant Appointments		
Date	Consultant	Outcome

Overview of Consultant Appointments		
Date	Consultant	Outcome

"It's All in Your Head"

At some point or another, *somebody* is going to tell you that it's all in your head. You might even be wondering that yourself. Hopefully my explanations regarding how our state-affiliated medical systems work will give some insight into how we might end up diagnosed with mental health conditions, but, just to make it clear, this is how that happens, step by step:

1. The results of the tests that consultants are allowed to give us are coming up clear, therefore, according to this system, there is nothing physically wrong with us.
2. Our symptoms mean that we tick lots of boxes that indicate mental health conditions, such as depression and anxiety.
3. In our state-provided medical system, depression and anxiety are treated with antidepressants and other medication.
4. If antidepressants and other mood-changing medications don't improve your physical health, they at least mean that you don't care as much about it.
5. You stop asking for help. You are cured. The problem must have been all in your head.

And there have been enough examples of this happening with complex illnesses for many, many years — ask anyone with ME/CFS or any other condition that our state-affiliated medical system can't "fix."

We all know that dealing with a vaccine injury has a huge impact on our mental health. Any complicated medical condition that isn't fully understood by healthcare professionals is scary. And this particular health condition is coming at a time where we are constantly triggered: our social media feeds are full of friends changing their profile pictures to joyfully indicate their vaccination status; our news sources are full of stories encouraging people to "get boosted now"; and, for some of us, we have not been allowed access to events and services unless we can prove that we are full vaccinated. We are *constantly* being triggered. If you weren't stressed/depressed/anxious before having an adverse reaction to the Covid vaccine, then you *sure as shit* will be afterward, especially given the current social climate.

Having a physical health problem that greatly impacts our mental health does not mean "it's all in your head." We need to be able to have useful conversations with medical professionals who might be the gatekeepers to us accessing other kinds of support. And that means being able to have a meaningful conversation with them about our mental health, if only to reassure them that it is something we are comfortable acknowledging and able to handle. Here's how to respond to doctors who tell you it's all in your head:

1. **Be calm.** Take a deep breath. Slow your heart rate. Remind yourself that you are safe. Protect your body while you respond. Stop your body from going into defensive mode because that's not good for your healing.

2. **Smile sweetly**, as if you really appreciate their kindness. Get ready to respond slowly — you are thinking carefully about their "diagnosis," so there's no rush. Again, take a deep breath.

3. **No temper or tears!** However hard it is, you need to control your emotional response as much as possible — otherwise, it will be perceived as validating their mental health comments.

4. **Agree with them.** Say something like, "I have no doubt that dealing with the impact the vaccine has had on my physical health has taken a huge toll on my mental health. It is sooooo kind of you to think about that." This keeps you calm, and clarifies that possible anxiety is a natural *symptom*, not a cause — it puts the word "kind" out there so both of you are reminded of the concept of kindness when dealing with each other.

5. **Reassure them.** Tell them what you've been doing to deal with your mental health. Say something like, "I recognised that too so I've been doing a lot of yoga/deep breathing/talking to my counsellor/writing/etc. I feel like I'm doing everything I can to manage my mental health and I know those things are working." This acknowledges what they have said and shows you are taking responsibility for the things you can do to help yourself.

6. **Ask for help.** Return the conversation to what you actually need help with by saying something like, "What I really need from you is support in dealing with my physical health, so how do you suggest we move forward with that?"

And always remember, regardless of what they say, you don't have to take their advice, and you don't have to speak to them again. If they won't support you in your recovery, move on and find someone who will.

Testing

Consultants can be very helpful in arranging for more complicated tests than those that your GP/PCP can arrange, but they do not provide the only way to get tested. You can arrange for your own testing through private practitioners or laboratories, and these tests do not require the cooperation of any medical practitioner, but they do carry a cost, and sometimes a very expensive one.

Keeping track of all the tests that you get done can be quite a challenge on its own. These two pages may help you organise your results.

My "Abnormal" Test Results			
Date	Test	Result	Further Action

My "Normal" Test Results			
Date	Test	Result	Rules out

Being Informed

It is not unusual for many of us to be more informed than our consultants about vaccine injuries, especially about those relating to the Covid vaccine. We have all seen a lack of knowledge among the healthcare professionals that we have turned to in the past and, more alarmingly, a lack of interest among those healthcare professionals to try to understand exactly what is going on with people like us. This lack of interest has resulted in many of us reading numerous scientific journals on Covid, Long Covid, vaccines, and the immune system, as well as countless other published articles on a variety of topics. Most of the medical professionals we have consulted with have not read the same articles that we have, and most of them are not aware of innovative, experimental treatments being conducted outside their field of expertise, medical system, or country. Until these new treatments are trialled in our own countries, we cannot expect to have a fruitful conversation with our consultants about them. We are more likely to find answers among our fellow vaccine-injured friends than we are among professional consultants ... for now.

Feeling Dependent on a Diagnosis

It can be very easy for us to become hyper-focused on the latest research and trying to get in front of one consultant or another, in the hope that they will be able to give us a definitive diagnosis, which in turn will mean we can start healing. Perhaps we need a different approach to consultants — perhaps we need to become less dependent on a diagnosis and more focused on healing. We can make healing a priority while still trying to get in front of specialists, but perhaps put a little less emotional investment in the latter. It takes a huge amount of effort (and sometimes money) to go through all the steps involved in accessing specialist support. That money and effort might be more helpful if it were invested in actual healing.

Just because we don't have a diagnosis or even any kind of consultant helping us, doesn't mean that we can't heal.

Wheel of Healing Update

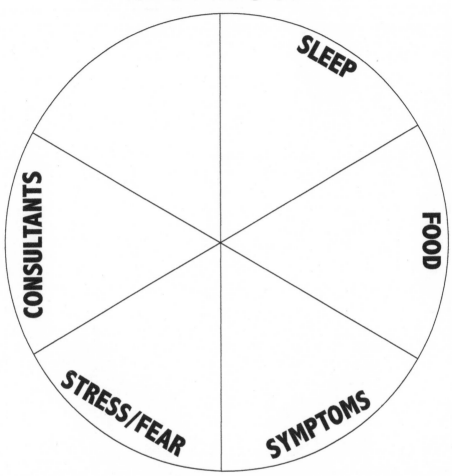

Before you add your actions regarding consultants, first take a moment to update your Sleep, Food, Symptoms, and Stress/Fear actions. How are you sleeping now? Does your diet need changing at all? Are you still motivated to follow it? What are your most problematic symptoms right now and how are you dealing with them?

Then, in the Consultants section, maybe add two things to focus on: perhaps try to focus on getting in front of a consultant who specialises in an area of health that is particularly bothering you. And maybe add one consultant who can support you with your full-body healing efforts. Don't try to add too many consultants — keep everything simple.

My Consultant Resources (names/websites/contact details)

Other Notes/Thoughts on Consultants

Before you start this chapter ...

Use the space above to make notes on the connections you have in your life. Who are the people closest to you? In which relationships do you invest emotional energy? How are those relationships maintained? What are the places or things that form your connections to the world? Some may have been made by choice, some may not. Some may make you feel good, and some may not. Take a bit of time to think about what the concept of "connections" means to you.

CHAPTER 6: CONNECTIONS

SUMMARY

Vaccine injuries are going to affect many of our relationships.
Not everyone is going to be supportive or even want to hear about it.
We need to be aware of those who will take advantage of our vulnerability.
We need to identify both helpful and harmful connections.
We can create our own safe space in the world moving forward.

Illness has a tendency to challenge the connections we have with the world outside our brains and bodies. Even something as simple as a cold can affect our interactions with friends, family, and colleagues. It might impact our relationships with social media, exercise, or time spent outdoors. It might affect our ability to do all the things that usually make us feel *joyfully* connected to the universe. We know this happens because we have felt ill before. We know we have to be patient. We know we will get over it. Feeling disconnected from everything about our normal lives is something most of us are able to cope with, *for a few days*.

Unlike a cold, illness from a vaccine injury lasts much longer than just a few days. If you're reading this book then you've probably already been dealing with it for a few months. Some of us have been living with it for a year and it's still ongoing. That's a long time to have your connections with the world disrupted. And because of the nature of this particular illness, there is another level of disruption to the connections that formed part of our lives before all this. The fact that our condition is related to a vaccine means that some of our connections aren't quite as full of empathy or compassion as we might have expected. And we may be surprised to find ourselves connected with new people specifically *because* we've had a vaccine. Not all of those connections are helpful, and some are even harmful.

The Vaccine Deniers

Scientists and researchers acknowledge that each one of us is complex, different, and unique in our physical, psychological, and emotional makeup. That's why part of the clinical trial stage for any medicine includes testing on a wide variety of people and *specifically* for the purpose of looking at adverse reactions. There may well be a lack of clarity around the number of adverse reactions, but the people who actually work in vaccine development do not claim adverse reactions are *nonexistent*. Yet we seem to regularly meet other people in our everyday lives who flatly deny that adverse reactions exist. And they can't wait to give us their opinions about people who say they are experiencing adverse reactions.

There are people out there who absolutely do not believe the vaccine is responsible for our health problems. You will come across them on the mainstream media, on your social media, during your medical appointments, and among your friends and family. Most of the ones you meet in person will at least be sensitive enough not to voice their denial (not to your face anyway), but you will meet with people who come up with all sorts of reasons to explain your ongoing health problems. They will propose *any excuse* except the vaccine itself.

If you feel you must respond to vaccine deniers, then you can quote some statistics from the vaccine manufacturers themselves; for example, "AstraZeneca state that very rare reactions occur in 1 in 10,000 people. Out of 52 million vaccinated people in the UK that's 5,200 experiencing adverse reactions. I guess I'm one of them." Then shrug it off like it's no big deal, and *move on*. Don't waste your energy.

How to deal with vaccine deniers? Don't. It is not your responsibility to persuade anybody to believe you. People who do not believe you are never going to be part of your recovery, and your recovery is your utmost priority right now. Vaccine deniers have no place in it. Whether they are a medical professional or a member of your family, *move on* from them. I have developed a personal rule: I do not discuss my health with any medical professional before ascertaining whether they are a vaccine denier or not. It's a waste of time for both of us. If it's someone close to me, then I either avoid the topic altogether, or accept that this is one of those times in life where I have a "relationship reshuffle," and someone that was once very important to me may not have a role to play in my healing. It's very difficult and there is some grieving involved. And the distance that grows between you because of this might be necessary for now, but it doesn't have to be forever.

The Vaccine Silencers

These are the people who do not deny that adverse reactions to vaccines exist, but are extremely uncomfortable with you talking about them. They say things like, "Yes, but we had to get back to normal somehow," or "Yes, but think of all the lives it's saved," or "Yes, but it's very rare," or, my personal favourite, "Yes, but if you talk about it you might put other people off having *their* jabs."

Vaccine silencers are much harder to deal with than vaccine deniers because the former are sending the message that the damage to your life is a sacrifice for the greater good. Somehow your pain is necessary. The fact that we're left in the lurch to deal with that physical and emotional pain doesn't seem to register with them.

They don't want you to tell them about your experience because it makes them afraid: afraid of what might be happening inside their own bodies, afraid of having their next jab, afraid that health professionals don't know what they're doing, afraid that the government or the media isn't sharing the whole truth, afraid of how we are going to move on with Covid, *afraid of not having control of their lives.* The vaccine-injured make vaccine silencers *afraid.*

People become defensive when they're afraid. They need reassurance that their experience, opinion, and world view is *right*, so that they can feel safe again. Vaccine silencers might be happy to talk about adverse reactions with you, but only for the purpose of convincing you to agree with them. They will ask you questions for the purpose of arguing, not for the purpose of learning. They are far more exhausting than vaccine deniers.

How to deal with vaccine silencers? Set your terms of engagement. State your boundaries, and stick to them. Identify on what terms you feel comfortable communicating with them, but know that you don't need to communicate with them at all if you don't want to. Again, you don't owe them any explanations.

My favourite way of dealing with them is to say, "I am willing to answer your questions, but for me this is a deeply traumatic experience that I am still living with, so I am not willing to argue with you." If all they want to do is argue and you make it clear that you will not participate in an argument, then they will lose interest in the conversation. But there is a chance that they will be happy to continue, and to learn a kinder way of communicating with someone who is vaccine-injured.

The "Vacurious"

I can't claim to have invented this fantastic word — my new friend Charlet (also vaccine injured) invented "vacurious" to describe people who have never had a Covid vaccine, have no intention of having one, but are obsessed with what the lives of vaccine-injured people are like. I would say that you will find these people online, but it would be more accurate to say that they will find *you* online.

Vacurious people are more exhausting than the vaccine deniers and vaccine silencers combined. If it is someone within your existing network, and they have just found out about your adverse reaction, they will think nothing of immediately contacting you to find out all the details about your vaccine injury, despite never having spoken to you in years (if at all). They have no comprehension of just how draining it might be for you to *again* go over everything that happened.

How to deal with the vacurious? Don't answer their calls, keep your texts or emails very short, and direct them to any social media or blog posts you may have made that explain what happened to you. The voyeuristic nature of the vacurious isn't going to be helpful in your recovery.

The Vaccine-Victim Saviours

These are the people who claim to be able to fix us. They present themselves as having all the answers — and such clear, simple ones — that they say they are using to treat "many" vaccine-injured people. Where all those magically recovered vaccine-injured people are isn't quite so clear, but the vaccine-victim saviours always have a website that bangs on about their miraculous cures and how you can purchase them. They portray themselves as the gatekeepers to those miracle cures, and do an incredibly effective job of convincing us that we should be following their guidance. They join our support groups, where they constantly post links until an admin works out that they're not vaccine-injured themselves and boots them out.

How to deal with vaccine-victim saviours? Accept that you are vulnerable right now, and that makes you prone to believe people who seem to be offering you hope. Nobody has any miracle cures for us. Nobody has any answers yet. If there were a miracle cure, then we would be talking about it among *ourselves*. It would be the only topic of conversation in our online support groups. There is no simple answer from any one individual that will make this all go away. Healing is a complicated, multi-layered process and nobody — however well intentioned — can "save" us. This vaccine-victim saviour complex is more about them than it is about us.

The Vaccine Vampires

These are the people that absolutely acknowledge that vaccine injuries exist and have probably been talking about what they see as the dangers of the Covid vaccine since our governments started talking about Covid. These people may have been very aware of adverse reactions to vaccines for many, many years. Of all the groups of people that we find ourselves connected with during this adverse reaction experience, this is the group that you'd expect would be greeting us with warmth, compassion, and kindness.

Not so. This lot are absolutely vicious.

Vaccine vampires stalk online media for tales of vaccine injuries. They take screenshots of our Facebook posts where we cheerfully announced getting our jab, then take screenshots of us in hospital a few days later, place the two photos next to each other, and then share them on their own social media. They attempt to infiltrate support groups to take screenshots of us talking about our symptoms, which they also then share on their social media pages. They collect stories in mainstream media of sudden deaths. There is a *gleeful* tone in their posts as they share stories of our misery. They are utterly toxic.

Vaccine vampires have lost their empathy and compassion to the extent that they will send hate mail to vaccine-injured people, tell us that we deserve the adverse reaction, and remove all the hope we may have worked so hard to nurture during our recovery. They truly believe that anyone who's had a Covid vaccine is going to die, and seem to take great pleasure in posting that "fact" in our support groups. It's a special kind of nastiness that very few people seem interested in protecting us from. If anybody in a cancer support group was there to just tell everyone in it that they were going to die, there would be *outrage!* Yet because we are vaccine-injured and nobody *really* wants to acknowledge our experience, vaccine vampires get away with it.

How to deal with vaccine vampires? You'll only ever come across them online because they'll never speak to your face, so report them. Then block them.

Dealing with Vaccine-Related Connections

Interactions with any of the aforementioned groups have the potential to trigger us both physically and emotionally, and often very unexpectedly. We are incredibly sensitive right now and any negative interactions can set us back days in our recovery, if not longer. But we can minimise the impact of unsympathetic or unkind interactions by being prepared and having ways of dealing with them at our fingertips. Remember the letter B when dealing with these connections.

The first B involves you sensing that the connection you have with that person feels a bit off. Are you thinking, "This is **b**ullshit," as you deal with them? If so, then you have the 3Bs to work with. You can:

1. simply **b**lock them (in non-online terms, walk away).
2. set a **b**oundary before you're willing to continue communicating.
3. have a come**b**ack at the ready.

Remember: Is this bullshit? How shall I respond? Block/boundary/comeback.

The chart on the next page might help you feel a little more empowered in your connections with unhelpful people, as well as give you space to play around with possible responses. Even if you don't use any of them, it always helps to offload or even just imagine how we would have liked to have responded to people who made us feel uncomfortable. Haven't we all walked away from a situation, only to then say to ourselves hours or days later, "I wish I'd said this instead?" Now you can reimagine that situation or be prepared for when it arises again.

I don't think other people quite understand how much their lack of empathy affects us. I have been quite shocked at people I had always considered to be very kind, who now communicate either online or in person in ways that I perceive to be very *un*kind, even cruel. This has been one of the biggest challenges of my having had an adverse reaction, and I had to find a much deeper and more healing way to cope with it — something more than the 3Bs can offer me. So now, after every connection with people like the ones listed on the next page, I remind myself that *most* people are doing what they truly believe is the best thing for humanity. It may be completely different from what I am doing, and from what you are doing, but that's OK. Even though it deeply hurt me when I first found out, I remind myself now that even the strangers who shared photos of my first trip to hospital believed that in doing so they may have been helping to save another person's life.

Vaccine-related connection	Connection name	My response (block/boundary/comeback)
Vaccine deniers		
Vaccine silencers		
Vacurious		
Vaccine-victim saviours		
Vaccine vampires		

Let's talk about the other connections we have — those that are not necessarily related to vaccine injury, but may play a helpful role in our healing from it.

Connection with Nature

So much about Covid (isolating and lockdowns are the obvious examples) has damaged our connection with nature. And if we're dealing with fatigue or paranoia as part of our adverse reaction, then that can also have a huge impact on our desire or ability to be outside. We all know that being surrounded by nature is good for us, and we need to make that a part of our ongoing healing, in whatever way we feel able. It might require significant effort. From spending time every single day on a beach or in a forest, wooded area, or garden, to just listening to a recording of a waterfall, and all the things in between, we need to spend time outside of our own thoughts and focused on something beautiful in nature, ideally while actually being out in it and breathing in fresh air.

Connections with Our Five Senses

Focusing on what we can see, hear, smell, taste, and touch is a common technique for dealing with anxiety, and something you may already be doing as part of managing the mental health impact of the vaccine on your life. This is something that we can all spend some time doing, every single day, perhaps multiple times a day if we feel we need to. We don't need to be anywhere specific and we don't need any special equipment. For example, right now I can take some time out from writing and spend a minute looking at the flowers painted on an antique kimono I have hanging on the wall, then a minute listening to the rain outside, then a minute smelling the fluffy hoodie I'm wearing because it smells like the neighbour's puppy I was cuddling earlier, then a minute drinking some hibiscus tea, then a minute running my hands over the Indonesian wood table I've got my laptop set up on, taking time to feel all the grooves, cracks, and knots. These connections with things outside my own head were vital in the early months of my recovery and, because the confidence I have in my own ability to cope with my situation ebbs and flows sometimes, I know that I would do well to employ this technique more often.

Connection with Our Sixth Sense

Our sixth sense — intuition or perception — can be our best friend or our worst enemy. It may become our worst enemy after an adverse reaction if, as for many of us, our sense of trust in the world has been fundamentally shattered because of this experience. We have discovered things about the world that mean we no longer trust a lot of what we trusted before. We may now be asking ourselves a lot of questions: Do we still trust our healthcare system? The doctors who work within it? The nurse who put the needle in my arm? The person who called to remind me to get a booster? Do we trust coroners? Do we really still "trust the science"? Do we trust our governments? Our police? The media? Many of us now find ourselves in a situation where we really don't know who or what to trust anymore. Add to that our bodies' ever-changing, unpredictable symptoms, and we don't know whether we can trust ourselves either — certainly not on a physical level.

All of the above affects our ability to trust, and this includes the trust we have in our psychological, emotional, and spiritual selves, which form a huge part of our intuition. And that intuition affects every other topic covered in this book: sleep, food, symptoms, stress, and consultants. Many of us find that our "sixth sense" is keeping us awake at night or has us worried about what food to eat. It can be on high alert either as a symptom in itself or as a contributing factor that slows down our recovery. Our sixth sense is anticipating every situation as potentially stressful, and second-guessing every interaction we have with consultants. Our sixth sense, or our intuition, is not helping us. It has, indeed, become our worst enemy.

Anyone who has ever been in an abusive relationship knows how that experience profoundly affects your intuition and general trust in the world. You lose faith in your own ability to judge whether someone is safe or not. You don't necessarily know what is a red flag and what isn't, so you go about your life fearful of making mistakes. Since we've returned to the idea of "fear," this may be helpful:
1. Revisit the Stress chapter, and specifically the part where you list your fears. Identify what your intuition is telling you to be afraid of during this time of uncertainty. Reacquaint yourself with the effects that "fear" has on your body, and use that knowledge as a motivating factor to put fear aside for a while.
2. Now also put your intuition aside. Just for a while. Tell it that you don't need it at the moment. Then decide not to either trust or mistrust anything. Take a break from your sixth sense.

Disconnecting from your intuition can be liberating. Reconnecting with your other senses can help you focus on the here and now. You can reconnect with your sixth sense later, when you feel the world is more deserving of your trust.

Connections with the Media

Of all the connections we've begun to question through this experience, the media is probably the one we're questioning most. All the different kinds of media seem to have a role within our recovery, so it's important for us to be comfortable with and purposeful about the connections we make with the media. We cannot passively absorb all the media we are exposed to because they have such massive potential to cause more damage to our health. We have to work out ways to protect ourselves from that. Because we know that the vast majority of media has its own agenda, we must establish boundaries.

- **Legacy media:** traditional TV, radio, and newspapers, and their accompanying digital platforms. These types of media have followed official government stances on Covid and the Covid vaccines. We tend not to see many stories about adverse reactions, and, if we do, such stories are preempted by statements about the benefits of vaccination.

- **New media:** podcasts, blogs, YouTube videos. These types of media are *in theory* independent but the platform upon which they are published may impose guidelines or warnings about potentially controversial content such as adverse reactions to the Covid vaccines or the vaccines themselves.

- **Social media:** Facebook, Instagram, Twitter, Telegram, and other platforms that encourage user interaction. Some are highly censored and users are removed for violating their guidelines. Some users posting potentially controversial content (such as information about adverse reactions to the Covid vaccines) are allowed to post, but their posts are hidden by the platform so that they don't automatically appear on someone else's feed (shadowbanning). Our support groups tend to be on social media, but are regularly shut down for violating guidelines.

When examining our connections with the media from the perspective of being vaccine-injured, we need to be aware that vaccine deniers, vaccine silencers, the vacurious, vaccine-victim saviours, and vaccine vampires are everywhere in the media. We have to be extremely aware of which media we consume, how much we emotionally invest in that particular media and its message, and how much time we spend consuming it. We need to constantly monitor ourselves in just how helpful or harmful that media is for our recovery. The next chart may be useful in this regard.

Media type	Harmful to my recovery	Helpful for my recovery	Healthy habits to work on
Legacy media (TV, radio, newspapers, and their digital platforms)			
New media (podcasts, blogs, YouTube videos)			
Social media (Facebook, Instagram, Twitter, Telegram, etc.)			

Connections with Support Groups

There are support groups on all social media, but they will be difficult to find on any *censored* social media, and they change all the time because they regularly get shut down by the platforms they are on. They may have names that don't spell out "Covid vaccine" or "adverse reaction," so it might not be obvious on first glance what they are. But keep looking. There are plenty of them and you will find lots of people dealing with the exact same challenges that you have.

There are usually quite strict rules for joining these support groups, and the admins work very hard to try to ensure that only actual vaccine-injured people get in (the vacurious and vaccine vampires love these groups), so sometimes applicants are misjudged. If your application to join inadvertently gets denied, just drop the admins a private message. Some groups will only allow you in with an invitation from an existing member. Most groups have a "reserve" group ready in case the original one gets shut down, so make sure you join that one too. And it's always a good idea to connect with a few active group members *outside* of the group so that you don't suddenly lose that feeling of connection provided by these support groups. They have quite literally been a lifeline for some people during their darkest hours.

A word of warning about support groups (and this is more about the time you spend on them than the nature of the groups themselves): it can be very, very easy to get drawn into constantly checking, commenting, or posting within the support groups. Our ability to manage the time and energy we invest in these support groups is just as relevant as our ability to manage the time and energy we invest in other media, if not more, because we *trust* our support groups. Know that everybody's circumstances are different — what works for one person might not work for you — and set yourself limits on how much time you're spending on the support groups. Set a limit to how many you join if that helps you manage your time better, and keep a strict eye on whether being in that group is helping or harming you.

My favourite support groups

Connections with Other Vaccine-Injured People

I've noticed that there are three kinds of people who are dealing with vaccine injuries, and you may recognise yourself here — maybe you've been all three of them at one point or another, depending on your stage of recovery. It is likely that you will connect with all three types.

First, there are people who seem to be stuck in that "panic" stage we were all at during the very early days when we started having an adverse reaction. These people are on multiple support groups and often post the same questions, repeatedly, over a significant period of time. They are having trouble getting to the first stage of recovery. They are having trouble accepting that this has happened and that there is any possible way forward. We have all been there and we all know what that stage feels like — perhaps this book has helped you move on from that stage yourself. These connections are a little tricky to manage — if you are further along the road to recovery, then of course you want to help, but you need to protect yourself a little too. You are still recover*ing*, and not fully recovered yet.

Second, there are vaccine-injured people who are very, very angry. Understandably so. Again, we have all been there, but spending too much time in anger or around someone who is angry is also not helpful for your recovery. You need to protect yourself a little when dealing with these people too.

But then there are some people out there who have handled their vaccine injury in a way that makes them a total inspiration. They are still recovering, but somehow finding the ability to share everything they are learning with others, to head up support groups, to speak out in a *kind* way to anyone who will listen, and to try their very best to smile through it all. These are the people you want to make your role models. Watch what they are doing — not what supplements they are taking or what diagnosis they have or don't have — watch how they are handling the entire experience. They will give you so much hope.

Vaccine-injured people who are my inspiration

Connections with Yourself

An adverse reaction to the Covid vaccine, in the middle of the global culture we are now living in, is a deeply, *deeply* distressing experience that disconnects us from everything that defined our world before this happened. Not only can it disconnect us from the world around us, but it can completely disconnect us from our sense of self. We may find ourselves asking all sorts of *big* and overwhelming questions, not just about our health and how we will be able to function again, but about our world and how it will be able to function again.

But more specifically, we may be asking ourselves, *how will we be able to function again within this changed world?*

How will we be able to function in a world that is so divided on the topic that we find ourselves right in the middle of? How do we move forward in a world that we have discovered is so dismissive toward those with vaccine injuries? How do we reconcile ourselves with the thought that there have been many, many people who have been injured by vaccines in the past, who we ourselves perhaps did not acknowledge or talk about? How do we talk about our experiences without intense conflict arising between us and people that we love deeply? How do we navigate our way through this world feeling that it is not a safe place for us to tell our truth?

I believe that we have to create that safe space ourselves. We have to create the world as we want it to be. We have to *be* that person we want to speak to ourselves. We have to change the language that we use to communicate with people who may not see the world as we do simply because they have experienced it differently. It doesn't matter if they aren't extending us the same courtesy — we are capable of creating the world we want to be in.

We have to create a bubble of safety around ourselves so that we feel able to speak our truth with a smile, set boundaries with firm kindness, meet an angry response with calmness, and understand that fear comes in many forms. We have to make a conscious decision to contribute to the world *as we wish it was*. We have to *be* the love and compassion that we wish we had received. We must surround ourselves with it.

That way we can be confident that the world will *always* be a safe space for us.

What does a safe space mean to me?	How can I create that safe space for myself and in the world in general?

Connections with Screens

At some point you'll have become aware that you are spending a lot of time staring at screens, especially on your phone, which is where we often connect with media, support groups, and individuals for both offering and gathering information. The addictive nature of screen use is not at all helpful for our healing. Also, in the early months of my adverse reaction, putting my phone anywhere near my ear resulted in excruciating pain — mobile phones are not conducive to our recovery. We need to impose strict limitations on the time we spend staring at them, or even being too close to them.

Connections with Government Representatives

Depending on your country, there are a number of government organisations or representatives that you'll need to connect with — this may not feel relevant in the early days but may be helpful further down the line.

If there are any vaccine compensation schemes in your country, then you should apply to them, even if you have no idea how long-lasting or permanent your health limitations will be. The earlier you apply, the sooner you may be given access to support. Likewise, if there are any government benefits that you may be entitled to, apply as soon as possible — don't wait for someone to tell you whether you're eligible or not. Just apply. Get the paperwork in as soon as you can. If you are self-employed, then don't assume that you are not eligible for government support.

Finally, write to your government representative. They are supposed to represent their constituents and, regardless of whether they actually do anything, you should at least have it on record as early as possible that you have notified them of your experience. They can be especially helpful if you are struggling to work your way around any government-organised compensation or benefits.

Connections with Advocacy Groups

At the time of writing, there is a "Post Vaccine Global Coalition" being established, which currently consists of 20 vaccine-injured individuals representing their countries and committed to advocating for recognition, research, and treatment for people living with adverse reactions to the Covid vaccine. The people within that group also run their own country-specific support groups. Advocacy for us is a very new development, and is one to keep an eye on.

Wheel of Healing Update

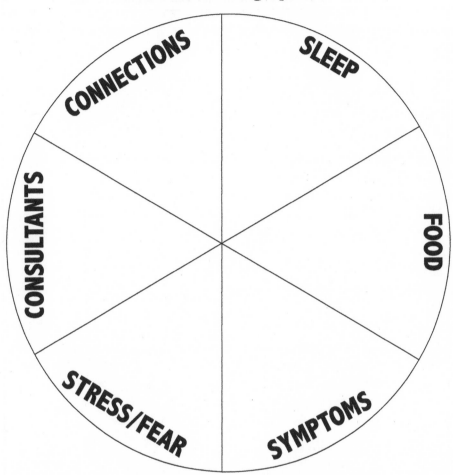

Before you add your actions regarding Connections, first take a moment to update your Sleep, Food, Symptoms, Stress/Fear, and Consultants actions. How are you sleeping now? Does your diet need changing at all? Are you still motivated to follow it? What are your most problematic symptoms right now and how are you dealing with them? Are there any new consultants you want to try to see?

Then, in the Connections section, make some notes on what you'd like to focus on. Do you want to withdraw from social media for a while? Is there a really uplifting podcast you'd like to listen to more regularly? Do you feel you need to be more connected to other people who are dealing with vaccine injuries?

My Resources on Connections (names/websites/contact details)

Other Notes/Thoughts on Connections

Wheel of Healing (spare)

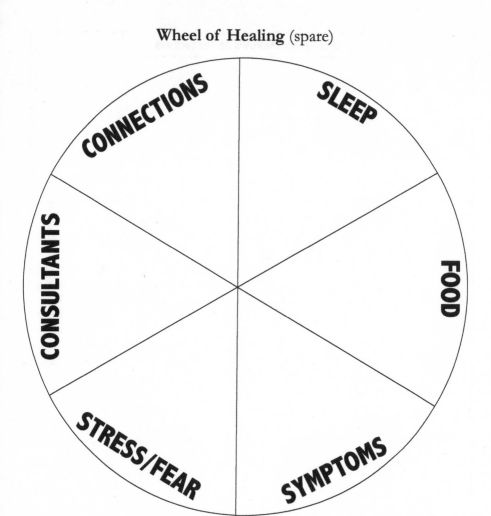

Wheel of Healing (spare)

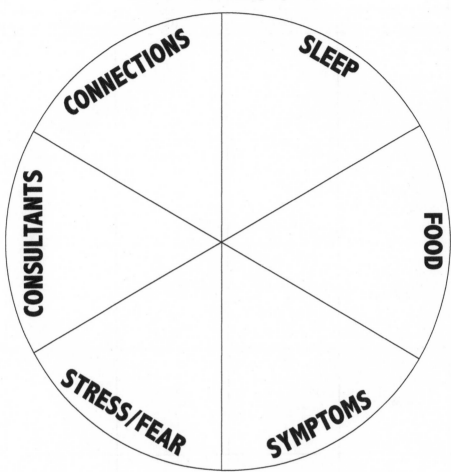

Weekly Diary			
	MON	TUE	WED
SLEEP			
FOOD			
SYMPTOMS			
STRESS/FEAR			
CONSULTANTS			
CONNECTIONS			

Weekly Diary (cont.)			
THU	FRI	SAT	SUN

Monthly Diary				
	Week 1	Week 2	Week 3	Week 4
SLEEP				
FOOD				
SYMPTOMS				
STRESS/FEAR				
CONSULTANTS				
CONNECTIONS				

Monthly Diary (spare)				
	Week 1	Week 2	Week 3	Week 4
SLEEP				
FOOD				
SYMPTOMS				
STRESS/FEAR				
CONSULTANTS				
CONNECTIONS				

Annual Diary						
	Month 1	Month 2	Month 3	Month 4	Month 5	Month 6
SLEEP						
FOOD						
SYMPTOMS						
STRESS/FEAR						
CONSULTANTS						
CONNECTIONS						

Annual Diary (cont.)						
Month 7	Month 8	Month 9	Month 10	Month 11	Month 12	NEXT!

ACCEPTANCE

I have personally felt that the concept of "acceptance" has played a key role in my own response to and ability to recover from what happened to me. Upon reflection, the most difficult times during the past twelve months have not only been when I've been dealing with the most debilitating of my symptoms, but when I've been trying to fight the experience the hardest. There were times when I was stuck in utter disbelief, and found it incredibly hard to simply accept what was happening to me. This was compounded by the difficulties I've had in accepting what's happening in the world in general, especially with regard to how vaccines and vaccine mandates seem to have affected the way individuals as well as governments are treating each other. Watching what has happened to the world during the past twelve months through the lens of a vaccine-injured person has, for me, been *immensely* distressing. I know that I am not alone in how I am feeling.

Some years ago I learned about empaths and their intense sensitivities to what other people are experiencing — we seem to feel others' pain even if we're not especially aware of feeling our own. I have noticed that there are many empaths among my new vaccine-injured friends, and I know that they have also struggled with what they see going on in the world in general.

I have noticed two other commonalities among many of my new friends — like many empaths, we have a history of trauma. That trauma is often abuse of some kind, but I can also see among us the kind of trauma that deeply distressing but non-abusive life experiences — like sudden bereavement — bring. I have also seen that some of us have already been subject to medical trauma and gaslighting prior to this experience. I have experienced multiple trauma myself, and learning about our bodies' response to trauma has been enlightening.

The other thing many of us can have in common is that we seem to be overachievers in life. Many of us were previously fit and healthy people — lots of us played sports or regularly exercised. Many of us were active members of our communities, we had busy social lives, and we were always on the go. We were multitaskers and our friends always commented on how full of energy we were.

Overachieving empaths with a history of trauma are undoubtedly going to find a serious health crisis incredibly difficult to accept. We are simply not wired to just *stop*. We are wired to keep fighting — it's how we have overcome all the other challenges that life has thrown at us before, yet still managed to create fulfilling lives that are productive and joyful.

Our tendency to fight may have served us very well in the past, but I do not think it will serve us well now. I have had to dig deep to find a way to do the opposite of what I would ordinarily do — I have had to find a way to accept everything that is going on in my body, and in the world.

I have had to accept that no one has any answers for me. I have had to accept that the people I thought would have been there for me, aren't. I have had to accept loss of friendship. I have had to accept that I may never return to working full-time again. I have had to accept that I may never run another 5K. I have had to accept that I really don't know how I'm going to feel from one day to the next. I've had to accept that this might be permanent. Or it might mean that time is up.

I have found reassurance in the acceptance of all those things. I still sometimes find myself "fighting" what is happening, and at those times my symptoms seem to become more bothersome — they are much easier to manage when I am at peace with them; when I move along through life as it is right now, allowing them to just be a part of the journey I currently find myself on. I hope to get to a point where this entire experience becomes part of what, for me, has been a rather eventful life — one full of wild and crazy experiences, but full of deeply loving and gentle experiences too. A life that I have always tried to fill with kindness, caring, and compassion for others.

I hope this book has helped you and that it continues to help you in finding your way to acceptance and the peace that it brings.

ACKNOWLEDGMENTS

Matthew, I will never *ever* be able to express my appreciation for everything you have done during this past year, and I am in tears just thinking about it. You saw the feisty woman you fell in love with five years ago fall completely apart. On multiple occasions, you have watched me get taken away in an ambulance without being permitted to accompany me. And you have watched me unable to so much as get out of bed for days at a time. You have fed me when I was unable to feed myself. You have kept the house *spotless*, for a year. You have provided a shoulder for me to lean on — both physically and mentally — throughout this whole experience, as well as offered that shoulder for me to cry on, over and over again. If it weren't for you, I would have lost my house, my business, and my sanity. I love and *appreciate* you so much.

Thank you to the friends and family who have supported us both during this past year. Thank you to all the people who have bought my books and my pickles in order to keep some level of income flowing in. Thank you to everyone that has kindly sent me links to one thing or another in the hope of providing useful information. Thank you to everyone that listened with kindness and compassion.

Thank you to Cathy, Melissa, Robyn, and Dr W — my healthcare team. You have all been incredible in your support and the efforts you have gone to in order to help me both cope and heal as much as I have. Robyn — your generosity and willingness to share so much of your knowledge with me has been a guiding light for me throughout this experience. You were the first person to give me hope.

And to my new friends around the world — my fellow vaccine-injured. Your strength and bravery keeps me going during the dark days. I love you all. Thank you for connecting with me, and for being so tolerant of my swearing. I've always had a potty mouth but it's got much, much worse since getting the vaccine. I think we may need to get it listed as a side effect in itself.

GET IN TOUCH

I would love to hear from you for any number of reasons:

- **Future editions:** If you have any comments, questions, or feedback you would like to see addressed in any future editions, please get in touch. Would you like to contribute to future editions yourself?
- **Other language editions:** Are you a translator who has found the English edition of this to be helpful and would like to get this out in your native language?
- **Other illness editions:** Does this book lend itself to another health condition that you're familiar with? Would you like to collaborate on a similar book?
- **More specific support:** Do you need more specific support, tailored to you? I have been informally providing some one-to-one support to individuals and, depending on my availability and capability, may be able to offer some level of personalised support.
- **Media:** Are you looking for someone media-savvy to interview about adverse reactions to a Covid vaccine?

I regularly write about ways that all of us (vaccinated or not, vaccine-injured or not, in agreement or otherwise) can emerge from these times with more compassion for one another. Find me on social media, or get in touch at caroline@carolinepover.com.

SUPPORT GROUPS

There are support groups for the Covid vaccine-injured all over the world but they are very hard to find. Due to censorship issues, group names are sometimes changed, group admins are sometimes suspended or banned altogether from social media, and groups themselves are sometimes shut down (which was one of the motivating factors for me to write this book). This is purely because of the nature of talking about vaccine injury on platforms like Facebook, Instagram, and YouTube, which have very strict guidelines. It can take a while to get used to the code in which we have to communicate online, so be patient. Twitter is more open to posts and comments about vaccine injury, and there are other fully open platforms such as Telegram, but Facebook is still the platform where most support groups have a presence.

It can be a little overwhelming when you first join these groups — the injured can be in very different places in their healing journey. Just take your time, know that people are all at different stages, and we are all different. What works for someone on that group may not work for you. And try not to spend *too* much of your life scrolling through.

The most comprehensive list of support groups is maintained at react19.org/international-coalition/. At the time of writing, there are groups in Australia, Belgium, Canada, France, Germany, Ireland, Israel, Italy, the Netherlands, New Zealand, Scotland, Spain, Switzerland, the Isle of Man, the UK, and the USA, as well as several international support groups such as React19, Real Not Rare, and Neuro V Long-Haulers. You are welcome to contact me if you're having trouble finding one.

I am a UK representative on the React19 Global Coalition, and a founding member of the support group UKCVFamily. UKCVFamily has an extremely active Facebook group, regular Zoom socials, and mainstream media campaigns. We offer GP letter-writing support and host online presentations by healthcare professionals. We also run an advocacy campaign where we will communicate with political representatives on behalf of any member, and we are legally represented in the UK's Covid-19 Public Inquiry. Please go to www.ukcvfamily.org to find out more.

You may have to search hard to find a support group but please know that we definitely exist, and when you find us, your life will completely change. You will no longer be alone.

BIOGRAPHY

Born in 1971, Caroline Pover grew up mainly in the south-west of England, and graduated with a First Class Honours degree from Exeter University before a desire for adventure took her to Tokyo in 1996, where she launched a number of community-focused businesses including her own publishing company. She lived full-time in Tokyo until the tsunami of 2011, after which she became heavily involved in supporting a remote fishing community in North-East Japan. Caroline raised £175,000 for them and managed over thirty different projects, while dividing her time between Japan and the UK. Based in The Cotswolds, she set up Auntie Caroline's — a gourmet pickle business supplying independent shops around the country and a regular feature in her local farmers' market.

Caroline has written a number of books, mostly related to Japan, including a book about the tsunami survivors, which won Best Memoir in the 2021 Next Generation Indie Book Awards. She has received numerous awards for her endeavours, including Plymouth's Top Ten Women of the Year, Japan-British Society Award for Contributions to Japanese-UK Relations, International Women's Day Outstanding Service Award, British Business Award for Best Entrepreneur, amongst others. She has given many speeches about her adventures over the years, including a TED Talk.

Caroline lives with Matthew and their two cavalier rescues in Cirencester. Having always had a keen interest in health, her adverse reaction to the Covid vaccine is currently taking her on another adventure.